"Heal Me or Kill Me"

My Road to Freedom from OCD

B.J. Condrey

Artwork (book cover) by Todd Goodwin of Revibe Media
(www.revibemedia.com)

DEDICATION

To Allison my wife, who makes me feel like I can change the world.

To my mom. Wow. What do I say? I need an entire chapter just to thank you for the role you played on my road to freedom. If not for you, there would be no dedication. There would be no book. There might not be a me. With all my heart, thanks for not telling me that I was stupid when you walked down the hallway that night. You turned the light on, both literally and metaphorically. I love you momma.

To every person who has suffered from Obsessive-Compulsive Disorder or loves someone who is suffering, this book is for you. Look up. There is hope! I wrote all of this for you.

TABLE OF CONTENTS

INTRODUCTION

A few months ago, I was asked to speak at my local church here in Picayune, Mississippi. In my message, I took some time to share a piece of my story concerning *Obsessive-Complusive Disorder* (OCD). Afterwards, an older gentleman came up to me and said, "I need to apologize to you. I have judged you in the past. I have always thought that you were not a genuine person, that you had not been through anything difficult, and that ultimately you were superficial." I think he was trying to compliment me. He sort of failed. Besides, what do you say to that? I do not believe the man was very wise for sharing this with me. That was between him and God. Why alert me to that issue in your heart? That being said, I understand what he was getting at. When a person digs down deep and shares his or her own particular story of pain, it becomes easier to identify with that individual. Do you have scars? Have you bled? Have you wept? My answer is yes.

I have *bled*.

I have *wept*.

I have felt *hopeless*.

This is not a self-help book. I hate those books. America's bookstores are full of them. Do you want your book to be read? Do you want to earn a living writing? Do you want people to know your name? Then write a book and title it something like:

Seven Steps to Satisfaction

Two Hops to Happiness

One Minute for Meaning

The Best Me That I Can Be

Ready to vomit? Good.

Americans tend to get excited about anything that promises world-altering transformation in three easy steps. Life usually does not work that way. Americans want to pull up to a spiritual drive-through, pay $5, and walk away a new person. Is this attractive? YES! Do I wish life worked this way? YES! Does it? Don't be stupid.

I suppose what I am trying to communicate is that, if you want a self-help book, please put this down and get your refund. It won't hurt my feelings. You will not find any 1-2-3 list. However, if you want hope, whether for yourself or someone you care about, then keep reading. As I constantly remind a young man that I am counseling right now in an effort to help him win in his fight with OCD, *this is the battle of a lifetime*. An inch of ground gained is worth celebrating. There are no quick fixes. To win the war, you have to start by winning a few battles.

So what do these pages contain? *My story.* And while I do stop at moments to discuss the nuts and bolts of OCD and to share a few comments along the way, this book tells the story of my freedom.

Freedom?

Yes, *freedom.*

Absolute freedom! Is that possible? Yes. I am living proof. Since age 26, I have been totally free of this mental illness. May these pages inspire you, give you hope, and deposit in your heart the truth that, with Jesus Christ, all things are possible. Freedom is possible. The life you see everyone living around you is possible. Imagine your most care-free day, a day not laced with OCD in any way whatsoever. *This is possible.* A care-free heart is free to wholeheartedly follow Christ and help others. Freed from self, you can engage. Desiring freedom is not selfish. Quite the contrary! A heart unchained from self can be poured out to anyone at any time. Only a free heart can respond to God's bidding upon any spontaneous prompting.

David wrote, "But You, O Lord, are a shield for me, my glory and the One who lifts up my head."[1] May the Lord do the work in you that He has done in me. I am so thankful. This book is my worship.[2] May it

---

[1] Psalms 3:3 NKJV

[2] The telling of any story, what we in the church label a "testimony," is proclaiming the work of God. By

3

be a fountain of hope in your life or the life of someone you know suffering from Obsessive-Compulsive Disorder.

---

declaring His works, we praise Him. So yes, this book is my worship!

"HEAL ME OR KILL ME"

*"Now I say very often - and people
don't like it - that God doesn't
answer prayer. He answers
desperate prayer!"*[3]

I was never officially diagnosed with *Obsessive-Complusive Disorder* (OCD). I'm not even sure there was a psychologist or psychiatrist in the little town where I was raised. However, I suffered greatly from this mental illness for years and years.

I grew up in a very small town in Northeast Texas. I had never heard of this mental illness. There was no *DSM-5* on our family bookshelf.[4] All I knew was that something horrible was wrong with me. I did not do it to myself. Nor did I choose it. This was truly an *illness*.

A *mental* illness.

As time marched forward, the illness grew. So did the hopelessness, the self-hatred, and a feeling of incompetence alongside swells of rage. Would the rest of my life look like this? Feel like this? Sound like this? Few thoughts are scarier to the human heart than the idea that the hell someone is walking

---

[3] Leonard Ravenhill. http://www.ravenhill.org/prayer.htm
[4] Granted, back then, it would not have been the 5th edition.

through may never end. When you start believing this, you are in deep, dark trouble. This is the sign hanging on the wall in Satan's lair. By the time high school rolled around, I was begging God for one of two things: *healing* or *death*. My prayer was simple:

"Heal me or kill me."

I was hurting, hopeless, and hated the taste of absolute bondage. I meant this prayer with all of my heart. The rest of the prayer went something like this:

"Lord, at this point, I do not care which. I would prefer to live. However, I would rather die than have to life like this the rest of my life. You have two options. Either heal me or kill me, and I am not interested in anything in between."

I meant it. Do not give me some *Mickey Mouse* version of Christianity. I had no time or interest for such a cheap commodity. People who are truly hurting never do. Either be God or end this absurd existence. No third option. Desperation produces such words. In the Old Testament, Rachel, grieved over her inability to bear children, once *shouted* to her husband Jacob, "Give me children, or I'll die!"[5] Patrick Henry, one of our founding fathers in America, once said, "I know not what course others may take, but as for me, give me liberty or give me

---

[5] Genesis 30:1

death!" Though he was speaking of *political* freedom, the cry of my heart was the same.

Thankfully, God chose the first of the two options I presented Him. He healed me, which is the reason you are now reading this book. I did not want to die. Yet, if that was the only way I could be free, then so be it.

You are probably thinking, "Why did I not commit suicide?" In *The Fellowship of the Ring,* Gandalf cautioned Frodo to not be so hasty in his desire to kill Gollum. He told Frodo, "Many that live deserve death. And some that die deserve life. Can you give it to them? Then do not be too eager to deal out death..."[6] I had a strong belief in the personal God of Christianity. I believed with all of my heart (as I still do) that only God can give life. Therefore, to take my own life, would be a gross and horrible sin. In some sense, I would be stealing, taking something that was not mine to take. The nature of my prayer should make more sense to you now. Morally, I did not feel I had the right to end my life. However, God was the one who gave me life, so He could take it if He so desired. Thus, I put the decision into His hands. If He was not going to heal me, then end my life. I could not, but He could.

To be honest, I did have many other things in my life that made me happy and brought me great joy

---

[6] J.R.R. Tolkien, *The Fellowship of the Ring* (New York: Houghton Mifflin Company, 1994), 58.

such as my family and sports. In the midst of the suffering, I still enjoyed certain parts of my life. But, there were moments this was not true. It was in these moments I prayed this prayer. I suppose that, like anybody struggling with anything, some days are horrible and some days are not. The prayers you pray depend on the particular day. All you need to know is that, even with all of the good in my life, I had many days that I prayed nothing but this prayer.

If you are a good pew-sitter, you may have problems with such a demanding prayer. Who am I to demand that the Creator, Sustainer, and Savior of the World bow to my command? Well, I will tell you who I am: *a son of God.*[7] His child. Sons and daughters are encouraged to "come boldly to the throne of grace" in order to "obtain mercy and find grace to help in time of need."[8] I was in too much psychological pain to mess with spiritual platitudes and formalities. I was dying on the inside. I did what I had to do. This was my *time of need.* Good people pray good prayers. Desperate people scream.

---

[7] I do not use this phrase lightly. In our day and age, phrases like this are thrown around a lot. The Bible teaches that though every human being is God's creation, NOT every human being is one of God's children. Rather, only the one who puts their trust in Jesus Christ and His work on the cross for the forgiveness of sins is a child of God. See John 1:12, John 14:6, and Acts 4:12.

[8] Hebrews 4:16 NKJV

I am convinced that this boldness was not irreverent. Rather, I hated my fear. I hated my anxiety. I hated my inability to function. I hated the way I always felt. And on top of it all, I was sitting in church every Sunday hearing about God's great power (and sometimes, even witnessing it manifested in the life of another).

Desperation breeds boldness.

God needed to do something, and I was getting to the point that even if death was the option He chose, at least it would mean relief. No one can suffer forever.

This struggle, however, is not where my story ends!

What happened?

God.

Jeffrey M. Schwartz, M.D., writes, "Simply defined, Obsessive-Compulsive Disorder is a lifelong disorder identified by two general groups of symptoms: obsessions and compulsions."[9] *Lifelong?* In most cases, this is true.

But this is not my story.

---

[9] Jeffrey Schwartz, *Brain Lock: Free Yourself from Obsessive-Compulsive Behavior* (New York: Regan Books, 1996), xiv.

Jesus Christ set me absolutely free. I do not live life striving to implement a set of cognitive-behavioral techniques in order to merely manage, or cope with, this illness. I am not on any medications. I am totally and absolutely free.

Sure, there are occasional moments when a tendency or two will surface, but that is all. It has no control or power over me. I dismiss them easily. Jesus Christ has completed such a thorough work of healing in my life that it is as if I never suffered from it in the first place.

Do not get me wrong, the road to freedom was a process. There were several critical points along the way. At times during the process, the illness seemed to get worse, not better. God did not wave some magic wand, speak some wizardly spell, and set my feet dancing. The path to freedom, even with Jesus Christ in the middle of it, was excruciatingly difficult and painful. I do not know why God did not heal me instantaneously. I wish He would have. I believe He can. But you know what? I do not care about that. All I care about is that once I was dead and now, I am alive!

The reality is that for some odd reason, God quite often moves slowly. *Very slowly.*

It is easy to become offended at God over such things. Why the delay? What purpose does it serve?

And yet, does Jesus Himself not say, "Blessed is he who is not offended because of me."[10] As my friend Thomas Lambert once spoke to a group of college students, "God is a crock-pot sort of God, not a microwave." In the end, freedom is worth the wait. The food and water came just in time. He heard my prayer. He did something about my suffering.

If you have OCD, you desperately need to read a story of some fellow traveler that found freedom. If you love someone that suffers from this mental illness, the anguish you feel coupled with the hopeless realization that you do not have the power to deliver them can be overwhelming. You need to read a story of hope as well. All throughout the book, I take time to share what you need to do in order to help the person in your life suffering from this illness. Whether you like it or not, you have a very significant role to play. Hopefully you will embrace this role. It was the difference-maker in my story.

The bottom line is this: *Jesus Christ can do for you what He did for me.*

So grab a cup of coffee, take a seat by a window somewhere, and dare to hope.

---

[10] Matthew 11:6

WHAT IS OBSESSIVE-COMPULSIVE DISORDER?

Hell.

A *mental* hell.

An *emotional* hell.

A death blow to your prayer life.

A relationship killer.

Tormenting.

All-consuming.

A fountain of hopelessness.

A source of rage.

A factory for self-hatred.

Paralyzing.

Unending anxiety.[11]

---

[11] "What is OCD," International OCD Foundation, accessed August 18, 2014, http://www.ocfoundation.org/whatisocd.aspx.

Obsessive-Compulsive Disorder is an "anxiety disorder in which the mind is flooded with persistent and uncontrollable thoughts and the individual is compelled to repeat certain acts again and again, causing significant distress and interference with everyday functioning." [12] The reason a person engages in such repetitive behavior is because that behavior is believed to be the sole means of alleviating the morbid anxiety resulting from the unwanted obsessions. A person will do anything for peace, right?

Before getting into the folds and wrinkles of my personal story, it is important to understand OCD from a "professional" angle. If you already have a solid grasp, then feel free to skip ahead to the next chapter.

* * * * * * *

What is an obsession?

Obsessions are defined as, "intrusive and recurring thoughts, impulses, and images that come unbidden to the mind and appear irrational and uncontrollable to the individual experiencing them." [13]

---

[12] Gerald Davison and John Neale, *Abnormal Psychology – 8th edition* (New York: John Wiley & Sons, Inc., 2001), 146.
[13] Davison and Neale, *Abnormal Psychology*, 146.

Obsessions may be *harmful, violent, immoral, sexually inappropriate, or sacrilegious.*[14]

Regarding obsessions, Dr. Schwartz writes the following: "The word *obsession* comes from the Latin word meaning 'to besiege'. And an obsessive thought is just that—a thought that besieges you and annoys the hell out of you."[15]

Whereas most people are able to recognize a thought at random and dismiss it, a person with OCD may feel guilty for a random thought. Why? These obsessions have an uncommon hold on people with OCD due to the fact that these thoughts are "frightening and torturous precisely because they are so antithetical to their values and beliefs."[16] This is one of the most powerful and insightful statements I have come across. One of the reasons that obsessions *feel* so horrible is because they suggest to the victimized person, "This is the real you." For this person, the fear becomes, "These thoughts would not be continually popping up in my mind unless they really are embedded in my heart. This must be who I am." This thought, which seems to be a moral indictment against the person, causes extreme distress and, in some cases, depression.

---

[14] "Pure Obsessional OCD (Pure O) – Symptoms and Treatment," OCD Center of Los Angeles, accessed August 18, 2014, http://www.ocdla.com/obsessionalOCD.html.
[15] Schwartz, *Brain Lock*, xiv.
[16] OCD Center of Los Angeles, "Pure Obsessional OCD (Pure O) – Symptoms and Treatment."

After all, to a person who deeply cares about the condition of his or her heart, this accusation is unnerving. For this reason, sometimes OCD can be worse in an individual who is deeply spiritual.

When an objectionable thought comes, a healthy person with a normal mind reasons, "Just because this thought entered my mind does not mean that it is *my* thought or desire. It might even be a temptation from Satan himself (this last thought applies to Christians who believe Satan to be a real presence and force)." A person with OCD assumes that if a thought entered the mind, he or she has automatically failed morally, or worse, if religious, sinned against a Holy God. This person fails to realize that it is not so much about what thoughts come into the mind. Instead, it is what you do with the thoughts that matter. The Bible says, "For we do not have a high priest who is unable to empathize with our weaknesses, but we have one who has been tempted in every way, just as we are---yet he did not sin."[17] God makes a distinction between *being tempted* and *committing a sin*. As long as you do not entertain the thought, you have not sinned. No moral wrong has been committed.

Whatever form the obsessions take, they transform even the ordinary, everyday tasks into over-whelming challenges. It can be exhausting. A person with OCD never gets an emotional break from the pain, anxiety, and struggle. It is so

---

[17] Hebrews 4:15

exhausting and can easily lead to an individual wondering at times if life is really worth the trouble.

* * * * * * *

What is a compulsion?

A compulsion is defined as, "a repetitive behavior or mental act that the person feels driven to perform in order to reduce the distress caused by obsessive thoughts or to prevent some calamity from occurring."[18]

Regarding compulsions, Dr. Schwartz writes, "Although a person with OCD usually recognizes that the urge to wash, check, touch things, or to repeat numbers is ridiculous and senseless, the feeling is so strong that *the untrained mind* becomes overwhelmed and the person with OCD gives in and performs the compulsive behavior." [19] The key phrase in this description is *the feeling is so strong.* For someone with OCD, life is reduced to the pursuit of temporal relief through any and all means necessary. If you have to hit a light switch 20 times, so be it. If you have to wash your hands 50 times a day, fine. If you have to touch anything with your right hand that you previously touched with your left to restore a sense of equilibrium, you do it. Don't argue. Don't fight it. Just give in because it

---

[18] Davison and Neale, *Abnormal Psychology*, 146.
[19] Schwartz, *Brain Lock*, xvi.

may very well be your only chance of dulling your conscience and quietening the powerful voices.

Consequently, you become a victim.

When you consider how many times you have to hit a switch, wash your hands, or turn a knob in a single day, this illness proves to be a death blow to normalcy. When a person begins to truly grasp just how much of life is being stolen, *rage* and *depression* often follow. Knowing that you are missing out on so much of what makes life meaningful and enjoyable (and at the same time feel completely helpless to do anything about it) can bring about an *existential* crisis. At this point, even suicide may appear a viable option. It is hard to keep putting one foot in front of the next when you lose heart.

* * * * * * *

OCD manifests itself in different ways. Dr. Allen Weg writes, "Like ice cream, OCD comes in different *flavors*."[20] Unlike ice cream, there are not any good flavors. Believe me, I tried several of them. Below is an *informal* glance at the varying types of Obsessive-Compulsive Disorder.

---

[20] Allen Weg, Ph.D., "The Many Flavors of OCD," *Living With OCD Blog,* July 16, 2011, accessed October 13, 2014, http://www.psychologytoday.com/blog/living-ocd/201107/the-many-flavors-ocd.

1. Checking
2. Contamination / Mental Contamination
3. Hoarding
4. Ruminations / Intrusive Thoughts[21]

The first type of OCD labeled *Checking* can be described as, "the need to check is the compulsion, the obsessive fear might be to prevent damage, fire, leaks or harm."[22] An example would be checking the knobs on an electrical stove over and over again because of the fear that one might burn the house down.[23]

The *Contamination* type of OCD comes in two different flavors (i.e., sub-types), one being physical and the other mental. The *physical* contamination sub-type of OCD can be described as follows: "The need to clean and wash is the compulsion, the obsessive fear is that something is contaminated and/or may cause illness, and ultimately death, to a loved one or oneself."[24]

The *mental* contamination sub-type of OCD can be described in the following manner:

---

[21] "The Different Types of Obsessive-Compulsive Disorder," OCD-UK, accessed October 13, 2014,
http://www.ocduk.org/types-ocd.
[22] OCD-UK, "The Different Types of Obsessive-Compulsive Disorder."
[23] OCD-UK, "The Different Types of Obsessive-Compulsive Disorder."
[24] OCD-UK, "The Different Types of Obsessive-Compulsive Disorder."

"It is almost as if they are made to feel like dirt, which creates a feeling of internal uncleanliness — even in the absence of any physical contact with a dangerous/dirty object. A distinctive feature of mental contamination is that the source is almost always human, unlike the contact contamination that is caused by physical contact with inanimate objects."[25]

A friend of mine that has also suffered immensely from this illness in the past shared that she at one point became terrified of acquiring cancer. She was overwhelmed with strong, powerful thoughts that if she got too close to someone with cancer, she might "catch" it. The cancer could "leap" from one person to another. In other words, she was afraid that she might be *contaminated.* Can you imagine really believing that cancer has the ability to leap-frog and how that would affect *every* aspect of your life? After all, you would never know who might have cancer whether you are at school, church, or the grocery store. I am guessing that after a while, you would have to end up staying away from anybody and everybody that you did not know very well in case they had cancer.

Hoarding is another type of OCD. This flavor of OCD consists of "the inability to discard useless or

---

[25] OCD-UK, "The Different Types of Obsessive-Compulsive Disorder."

worn out possessions, commonly referred to as 'hoarding'."[26] Of all the flavors of OCD, I am least familiar with this kind. I have never personally come into contact with anyone suffering from this type.

The last major type of OCD is labeled as *Ruminations / Intrusive Thoughts*. A rumination is "a train of prolonged thinking about a question or theme that is undirected and unproductive."[27] These can include important life questions as well as philosophical questions. This is a little tricky. After all, part of what it means to be human is to ask, search out, wrestle with, and form conclusions in response to important questions. I suppose the difference between a normal person asking such questions and a person with OCD asking these questions is that the latter is severely impaired in everyday life from such questioning. Again, this might be a fine line. People throughout history have had seasons when one felt unable to go on with life because of a sense of meaninglessness.

Under this last heading, *intrusive thoughts* are also mentioned. Intrusive thoughts can be defined as, "obsessional thoughts that are repetitive, disturbing

---

[26] OCD-UK, "The Different Types of Obsessive-Compulsive Disorder."
[27] OCD-UK, "The Different Types of Obsessive-Compulsive Disorder."

and often horrific and repugnant in nature."[28] Sexual thoughts are *one* example and cause inexpressible distress.[29] One sub-type of this kind of OCD is known as *Pedophile OCD.*

Monnica Williams, Ph.D., shares the following story from her own experience:

> *"I have an inpatient who worries that he might be a pedophile," the psychiatrist said. "I think it's OCD, but he has a young daughter and our social worker wonders if we should make a report to children's services." This was when I first heard about "John," as we'll call him. A psychiatrist at a local hospital contacted me because he wanted to consult about their latest admission. The treatment team was divided on his diagnosis and what the next steps should be.*
>
> *John was a devout Christian, tormented by unrelenting thoughts that he was really a child molester – a ticking bomb just waiting to go off and cause harm to his young daughter, her friends, and any children he might get his hands on. These terrifying thoughts became so upsetting that John fell into a deep depression, finally*

---

[28] OCD-UK, "The Different Types of Obsessive-Compulsive Disorder."
[29] OCD-UK, "The Different Types of Obsessive-Compulsive Disorder."

contemplating suicide as the only way to keep his daughter safe. That was when his family took him to the ER...

"Whatever you do, don't make a report until I have a chance to asses the patient," I told the psychiatrist. I knew that if John had OCD, it was very likely that his form of the disorder would not be quickly understood by authorities, potentially resulting a stressful quagmire of legal issues surrounding his ability to be a parent. That sort of added stress would be the very thing that might drive an already fragile person over the edge. It is true that John was in no shape to function in any capacity, much less as a father. He had been demoted at work due to his condition, as he was frequently distracted, or he would call in sick due to depression. However, people with pedophile OCD (or POCD, as it is sometimes called in the online OCD communities), are actually the least likely to harm a child. In fact, John cared so much about the well-being of his daughter that he was willing to kill himself to keep her safe.

After John was discharged, I conducted a comprehensive assessment of his symptoms. He had been diagnosed with OCD at age 12. He used to worry about religious and spiritual matters, like if he was going to heaven after he died, but as he got older his worries shifted into other areas. He once feared that he might be attracted to his sister, then that he might be gay, and most recently that he might be a pedophile...

It's important to understand that John was never attracted to children (nor men, nor his sister). OCD is a malfunction in the brain that causes catastrophic worries about things that are very unlikely to occur...

By the end of the treatment program, he was feeling tremendously better...John became convinced he was not a pedophile.

I am always amazed by how quickly this treatment can help people get their lives back, which is one of the reasons I love working with people who have OCD. John was able to resume his normal life after just 17 sessions. In fact, he remains so grateful and excited about his recovery that he was willing to share his experience on a local TV show, The Power to Change.[30]

I admit that this story is a little lengthy. However, if you do not have OCD or have never had contact with anyone who does, this story can help you grasp, at least cognitively, how this illness works

---

[30] Monnica Williams, Ph.D., "Could I Be a Pedophile? The Worst Kind of OCD," *Culturally Speaking Blog*, December 25, 2012, accessed October 13, 2014, http://www.psychologytoday.com/blog/culturally-speaking/201212/could-i-be-pedophile-the-worst-kind-ocd.

and how destructive it can be. This illness is difficult to understand. The natural tendency for a person who has not had any exposure to someone affected by OCD is to dismiss the entire ordeal as something stupid that can be overcome at any moment with a good dose of will power. You need to understand, it is much more powerful than that. The worst thing you can do if in contact with someone suffering with OCD is minimize their struggle and dismiss their suffering. It is that real. It is that dark.

As Dr. Williams points out, "This is the paradox of OCD. It takes the very thing a person cares the most about and turns it upside-down."[31] If you care about sexual purity, this might in fact be the one area that obsessional thoughts hit you the hardest as in the case of John. This is a sad and heart-breaking phenomenon. If you are connected with someone suffering from this mental illness, please do not give up on the person. Try your best to understand. Listen with tenderness. Do not judge. No matter how helpless or frustrated you may feel at times, continue to show compassion. The person needs kindness. Be an alternative voice from what they hear every day in their own head. Your kindness, tenderness, truth, and compassion may be the only thing standing between them and an eventual suicide.

---

[31] Williams, "Could I Be a Pedophile? The Worst Kind of OCD."

Remember, it is not your job to "fix" your loved one. Not only is it not your job, you cannot do it if you tried. Only God can change a person's heart. Only God can rewire someone at the deepest level. If the person with this mental illness senses that you are trying to swoop in and "fix" them, it is over. You have lost the individual. He or she will no longer confide in you. You are no longer a safe place. I believe one of the reasons for this is that when someone tries to "fix" us, our natural response is to believe that the person trying to help does not understand what we are really going through. If they did, they would not think the problem could be so easily solved. To suggest the problem can be solved in such an effortless manner implies that one does not understand the extent to which the person with OCD suffers. Besides, many of us go around trying to fix people for no other reason than we are frustrated and want that person to get over it. Our "fixing" ceased to be about the *other* long ago. A person can read right through this attitude.

Though much more could be said regarding these four types of OCD and their corresponding sub-types, the above information is adequate to show just how many flavors of OCD there are. There are vast amounts of material that you can go to in order to acquire a better understanding of this mental illness. For my purposes, this suffices.

THE ORIGIN OF *MY* OCD

"Rome wasn't built in a day."

Last chapter, I treated OCD in more of a classroom style. It can be helpful to understand the nuts and bolts of OCD. Granted, there is nothing magical about information. However, knowing what you are up against or what someone you love is up against can be of great benefit.

Though a generic understanding of this illness is important, it is not why I wrote the book. If you are suffering with OCD or are hurting because someone you love is suffering from this illness, what you really need is for someone to pull up a chair, take your hand, look you in the eye, and hold nothing back.

There is no substitute for vulnerability.

I wrote this book to do just that, that is, to be transparent. A lack of transparency would leave a bad taste in your mouth. The book would read more like a *textbook* than a *story*. Textbooks inform us. Stories change us. I want you to know just how bad I suffered at the hands of OCD so that you will not be tempted with the thought, "Well, the only reason God was able to set him free is that his version of OCD was not that bad." After all, there is nothing impressive about snapping a twig in-between your fingers. Anybody can do that. God is not needed. But a chain? That is impressive. I want you to see how thick my chain was so that faith will sprout in your heart. A candle shines brightest in a dark room.

* * * * * * *

Small events can, over time, produce gigantic ripples.

When I was around seven years of age, the OCD began. Its beginning was small. Seemingly out of nowhere, I found myself trying really, really hard to avoid stepping on any and all sidewalk cracks. As a child, I had no knowledge of OCD, so in my mind, there was not much harm to what I was doing. On the other hand, it did not feel like all of the other games I played. Other games were fun, spontaneous, and exciting. This "game" seemed much more serious. I felt like I *had* to play this game.

The game went like this: *Any time I was walking on a sidewalk, I would continually whisper to myself, "If you step on a crack, you will die."* If I remember correctly, sometimes I would tell myself that my mom would die if I stepped on a crack. Because of how much I loved my mom, this no doubt raised the stakes. A crack was my enemy. The pressure was real. I could not mess up.

One person who suffered with OCD confessed,

"Getting dressed in the morning was tough, because I had a routine, and if I didn't follow the routine, I'd get anxious and would have to get dressed again. I always worried that if I didn't do something, my parents were going to die. I'd have these terrible thoughts of harming my parents. I knew that was completely irrational, but the thoughts triggered more anxiety and more senseless behavior.[32]

When walking on pavement, I was engaged in a life-or-death activity. I recognized that this thought was irrational. However, my feelings spoke much louder than my reason. One characteristic of OCD is that no matter how irrational the belief may be, it is accompanied by a miserable, anxious, fearful web of emotions. In other words, the threat might as well be real. The thoughts and emotions are simply too strong to be able to do what normal people do, that is, recognize the ludicrous nature of the thought and thereby dismiss it. Simply stated, it is not that easy for a person suffering with OCD. In addition, what makes it worse is that friends and family members often consider OCD to be some stupid problem that the person could throw away like a bad shirt if one

---

[32] "Introduction: Obsessive-Compulsive Disorder," National Institute of Mental Health, last modified 2013, accessed October 13, 2014, http://www.nimh.nih.gov/health/publications/obsessive-compulsive-disorder-when-unwanted-thoughts-take-over/index.shtml.

wanted. The implicit message in this type of response is that the only reason you still have this is because you will not let go. It is that easy. This attitude quite often leads the friend or family member to respond to the suffering individual's repetitive behavior (or set of behaviors) with a flippant, "Well, just stop doing that," whatever *that* may be. This of course results in the OCD person feeling even less understood and more hopeless than before. It is no secret that one of the loneliest experiences in life is when you feel like no one, especially those closest to you, understands what you are going through. My mom was the first to understand me. She was the first to give me hope. If you are close to someone who has OCD, please pay attention. She rescued me. She saved me. I was drowning, and she kept me afloat until God sent a ship to carry me to the shores of freedom. Her understanding and compassion *alone* was enough to help me get the oxygen I needed to stay alive. She bought me time. I love you, mom. Thank you.[33]

This was my OCD's small beginning. Cracks in the sidewalk. Life or death hanging in the balance. Over time, it became all-consuming. In case you haven't noticed, there are cracks in the sidewalk every few feet, and if the sidewalk is old and there are tree roots around, you can multiply the number of cracks exponentially. To cope, I developed what I now call, *step-timing.* To try and reduce how much these

---

[33] The specifics of the role my mom played are forthcoming in later chapters.

sidewalk-obsessions dominated my life, I did my best to establish a rhythm to walking so that with minimal mental effort, I could miss the cracks without having to try so hard to do so. And somehow, I would do all of this while living life and walking alongside people. I was always in two worlds, one on the outside, one on the inside. Externally, I wanted people to think I was normal and did not want to let on that something very strange was happening. Internally, I was performing elaborate mental and emotional gymnastics in an effort to regulate my behavior in such a way that I could enjoy some morsel of peace.

Though I was very young, the seeds had been planted. Brokenness had been set into motion. It was just a matter of time.

MY PRE-TEEN AND TEENAGE YEARS

*"For if you remain silent, I will be
like those who go down to the pit."*[34]

As if being a teenager is not challenging enough, my pre-teen and teenage years are when my OCD came to full fruition. It took over. Though I had so many other wonderful things going for me, all took a backseat to this struggle. I was winning regional and state awards in high school basketball, had the most amazing family ever, was working toward being 3rd in my class, had a good job, and had a vehicle given to me from my grandparents. Yet, in the midst of all of this, there were moments I felt so dominated, controlled, and oppressed by the OCD. It was sucking the life right out of me.

* * * * * * *

Around the age 10, one minor way that my OCD manifested itself was in church. During the service, I would interlock my fingers. But, in some inexplicable sense, I felt as though I was not able to interlock them a "perfect" way. So, I would push my interlocked fingers together harder and harder, messing up the blood circulation in my hands. At this point, it would be evident by the red and white

---

[34] Psalms 28:1 (last part of verse)

splotches on my hands how hard I was pressing my fingers together. There were moments I felt as though I had got my fingers into a perfect position. That never lasted long. Any peace was short-lived. For the most part, I could never get my fingers interlocked in such a way that I felt good on the inside. There was one moment I was so caught up in my own world performing this particular behavior that I did not notice my mom watching. She said something to me after church but did not think anything more of it at that time.

As is characteristic of OCD, the feeling of not being able to perform some task perfectly was emotionally disturbing, even with something as insignificant and stupid as not being able to interlock my fingers in just the right way. I could not attain perfection and this drove me crazy.

* * * * * * *

Another way that the OCD manifested itself in my life was with switches, especially light switches. This was one of the most horrible, tormenting areas for me personally. Remember, every person's OCD looks a little different than someone else's. *Switches* were my hell.

At eight years old, I prayed and asked Jesus Christ to come into my heart and life, forgive me of my sins, and be my Lord. Due to this conversion, I had, even at a young age, an intense desire for purity and holiness. I wanted to have a clean mind and a pure heart. Did the Bible not say, "Blessed are the pure in heart, for they will see God"?[35] Or, "Who may ascend the mountain of the Lord? Who may stand in his holy place? The one who has clean hands and a pure heart..."[36] I wanted everything about my life to please The Lord. David once wrote, "Create in me a clean heart, O God."[37] This was my desire as well, to be "fully pleasing [to] him."[38]

Like anything good, Satan can corrupt it. He can take something originally wonderful and beautiful and, with great perverting powers, color that good thing in such a way that it actually begins working against you rather than for you.

This is exactly what he did with my desire for purity and holiness. Satan took this wonderful, divine desire in my heart, and started lying to me about what purity and holiness really meant. Once the lie was embedded into my thinking, it was easy for him to lead me down a dark path. Let me explain.

When a bad thought comes to mind, you have not yet sinned. If you are not clear on this, you do not stand a chance of living free of guilt and condemnation. After all, who can control what thoughts come at you on any given day? Just because you think a thought, this does not mean you

---

[35] Matthew 5:8
[36] Psalms 24:3-4a
[37] Psalms 51:10
[38] Colossians 1:10 NKJV

have sinned. When a thought appears, whether lustful, angry, hateful, or envious, what you do with the thought immediately following its appearance determines whether or not you sin. If you let it hang around for a while, you have sinned. If you discard the thought quickly, you have not. Our thoughts matter to God. Our thought-life is of the utmost importance to the Lord.

This line of demarcation between temptation and sin has not always been so clear. As a teenager, I had an intense craving to live righteously. Though involved in high school athletics and being very popular in school due to my success in basketball, I made a point to never cuss. I felt that as an athlete, I could show people how different I was by not using foul language. My heart's desire was that once they noticed this difference, it would not be long until they discovered what it was that made me so different—*Jesus Christ lived in me*.

Satan, however, perverted this good desire in my heart. It was so important to me not to cuss that the OCD begin to feed off this desire. If I were to tell you not to think about a pink elephant for the next 30 seconds, good luck! Right? The more you try not to think about something, the harder it is to not think about that particular item. It was the same for me. My enemy knew this. He played off the good desires in my heart as well as a heightened sensitivity to guilt. Anytime I would go to flip the light switch on or off, a cuss word would enter my mind. Normally, a person would dismiss this as a random thought, maybe a temptation, nothing more. Walk away and let the thought go. It was not that easy for me. I would experience a deep sense of shame that I could not flip a switch without a dirty word entering my mind. I was defiled. Something was wrong with me. I knew it.

Looking back, it seems so silly. Who cares about the cuss word in my head, right? These days, I would laugh it off. God does not care about what randomly enters my thoughts. Rather, He cares about how I handle those thoughts. I know that now.

In these moments, a gnawing, screeching guilt would demand that I flip the switch back to its original position and try again. Now for a second time, I must attempt to flip the switch without a cuss word entering my mind. The pink elephant grew larger. The harder I tried to keep a bad thought out of my mind, the more difficult it became. It is virtually impossible to simultaneously flip a switch without thinking of a cuss word while telling yourself not to think of a cuss word. The sheer fact that I was telling myself not to think of a cuss word was enough to keep cuss words in my head. Every time I flipped the switch and a cuss word surfaced, I had to start over. Ten times. Fifteen times. Twenty times. Until either I somehow accomplished the impossible feat, or, until I heard somebody coming toward my room. In the case of the latter, I did not want to get caught. The problem was that though the sound of someone coming was enough to make me stop (in order not to be found out), this by no means meant that the emotional storm had passed. Sometimes it became worse. After all, I had not flipped the switch in the "right" way. I had not satisfied the perfect standard. The internal crisis had not been resolved.

I would walk away out of fear of being discovered though my emotions would continually scream at me because I had not resolved the situation. I would sometimes go back. Until I went back and was able to flip the switch in the "right" way, my emotions would torment me. They were so loud, so aggressive, so penetrating. I was miserable and discouraged. I honestly could not imagine there being another person in the world that was so terribly stupid and pathetic as I. Who could not stop flipping a switch? What a joke. I was the joke.

If you have never suffered with OCD, you may be asking yourself, "What does it even mean to speak of flipping a switch in a 'right' or 'perfect' way?" But that is exactly my point. That is how overwhelmingly powerful obsessions can be. I truly felt as if I was guilty of a significant moral and spiritual failure if I could not flip the switch at least once without a "dirty" thought coming to mind. The more I tried, the angrier I got. Imagine being in a prison cell, hating it with every ounce of your being, seeing that the door to freedom is open, and still, for some strange reason, not being able to get through the door though you are screaming for it with your whole heart. Feelings of bitter rage would eat up my heart as I stood there trapped in these insanely irrational situations. I knew the problem was with me. I hated me. I raged at me. There are no words to communicate the volume of self-hatred I experienced realizing how something so irrational was both controlling and destroying any chance I had for a normal existence.

I did not struggle with just light switches. Door knobs, car door handles, a/c dials on my car dash, and all of the buttons and dials on my aftermarket CD player posed similar challenges. Now, how many times a day are you flipping switches, getting in and out of your car, and turning knobs and adjusting the temperature? It would be impossible to keep count. Everywhere I turned there was another knob or another switch. This part of the OCD was truly one of the most difficult for me to handle. As described, it was all consuming. Life was quickly becoming nothing more than a collection of obstacles.

I was losing heart. I was falling short. I could not meet the standard.

* * * * * * *

Another way that OCD stole from me during my teenage years (and after) was in my prayer life. I am convinced that OCD is not only a biological and psychological phenomenon, but also spiritual. There is no doubt in my mind that there is a strong, spiritual component to OCD.

I consider it more than coincidence that OCD severely frustrated my prayer life. I remember lying on my bed at night trying to pray before I went asleep. As in all other areas of OCD, my prayers never felt up to par. I could not pray perfect enough. This was not God's opinion, but at the time, I believed it was. The negative, nagging feelings of disapproval were so loud that no other thought was able to penetrate my fortress of lies. I was held captive. I really believed that I was praying prayers that Jesus hated. They were not good enough. I was not good enough. I needed help from something or someone on the outside. I could not escape the idea that God despised me. As a result, I felt a piercing disgust with myself. Who can be at peace with himself if he feels that he is not at peace with God? The line between perception and reality was blurred. It was all the same. I could no longer differentiate between the two.

In a Biblical, Christian worldview, God has an enemy. His name is Satan. It is a travesty that in America, the devil has been "cartooned" out of our understanding of reality. For the most part, people do not have a problem believing in God (even if our idea of God varies widely), but people are discarding the belief in a devil. This day and age, if you really believe in Satan, you are considered a naive simpleton, one who refuses to embrace a more intelligent, sophisticated worldview.

I believe that your faith and life will be a poor expression of what Jesus Christ intends if your worldview does not include the reality and presence of Satan. Jesus once said, "The thief does not come except to steal, and to kill, and to destroy. I have come that they may have life, and that they may have it more abundantly."[39] God is wholly good and Satan is wholly evil, and though the war has been decided, smaller battles are being waged every day. And take note: By *smaller*, I in no way whatsoever mean *insignificant*.

The ultimate war being fought is for the souls of men and women. Will each person spend an eternity in Heaven or Hell? Will a person be forever separated from the love and kindness found only in the presence of God? As important as this is, when Satan loses this ultimate war, he does not entirely give up. There are still other battles to win.

C.S. Lewis' book, *The Screwtape Letters*, is a "recording" of a conversation between a high ranking demon named *Screwtape* and a lower ranking demon named *Wormwood*. Wormwood is assigned to a particular human being. Despite all of his efforts, the human he is assigned to chooses to follow Christ. Upon hearing this, the high-ranking Screwtape informs Wormwood, "I note with grave displeasure that your patient has become a Christian. Do not indulge the hope that you will

---

[39] John 10:10

escape the usual penalties..."[40] Following this sharp rebuke, Screwtape goes on to tell Wormwood, "There is no need to despair; hundreds of these adult converts have been reclaimed after a brief sojourn in the Enemy's[41] camp and are now with us. All the *habits* of the patient, both mental and bodily, are still in our favor."[42] In this fictitious but all-too-real dialogue between these two demons, Hell still held out hope that though a decision had been made for Christ, there were still many battles that could be won. If Satan cannot keep you from Christ, he will settle for keeping you from walking in the fullness of Christ. A *lame* Christian is still something he takes pride in.

Though Satan had lost the war of eternity concerning my life, he piggy-backed on my OCD and, through it, wreaked havoc in my relationship with the Lord. He had me convinced that my prayers were lousy and pathetic. Thus, I would repeat words, phrases, and sentences over and over. I was miserable. Emotionally, it was the exact same experience I had when flipping switches. No matter how hard I tried, I could not do it "right." My options were twofold: Either stop praying or keep repeating myself (just like the switch) until I prayed in a manner that *felt* correct. My version of OCD

---

[40] C.S. Lewis, *The Screwtape Letters* (San Francisco, HarperSanFrancisco, 2001), 5.

[41] "Enemy" here is actually referring to God. Remember, this is Satan's servants speaking.

[42] C.S. Lewis, *The Screwtape Letters*, 5.

was interlaced with an exorbitant amount of perfectionism. It was killing me from the inside out. I loved God and wanted my relationship with Him to grow. However, when it came to the very activity that enhances intimacy (i.e. prayer), I once again felt like I came up short. Once again, a *failure*. I didn't have what it takes.

I am not prepared to say that my OCD was actually from Satan. After all, there is much I do not know. Was a spirit of fear ministering to me? Another kind of spirit? Was this primarily psychological with spiritual undertones? Whatever the case may be, I am sure that the enemy of my soul was quick to use OCD to further his purposes in my life. You can be sure that one of his main purposes is to block your intimacy with God at all costs. If he is successful in doing this, hundreds of other victories (for Satan, *defeats* for you) will follow. In the Christian life, our every movement and motivation is to flow out of intimacy with God. Satan was killing my heart by keeping me from simple, authentic prayer. No matter how hard I tried to pray, it just got worse. My prayer life was reduced to nothing more than trying to say something in just the right way. When prayer becomes this performance-based, you may keep trying, but, over time, you grow to despise it.

I was losing heart. I was falling short. I could not meet the standard.

* * * * * * *

41

Another outgrowth of my OCD was this constant, internal demand to both establish and maintain *psychological symmetry*. The moment I felt *emotionally* off-balance, the situation had to be remedied. For me, this was one of the areas that OCD struck me the most. This is best explained using examples.

Pretend I am about to go to bed. I pull out the dresser drawer to retrieve an item with my left hand. I then close the drawer. At this point, the normal person would lie down and go to sleep. But, not me. Not back then. I would, in a way difficult to explain, feel extremely off-balance. I had just opened and closed the drawer with my left hand. It was as if something was now in my left hand that was not in my right. To counter the extremely unpleasant feeling of being off-balance, I now needed to mimic my left hand's behavior with my right hand. To reestablish this intuitive, emotional equilibrium, I with my right hand would open the same dresser drawer and then close it. All should be good now, right? What I had done with my left hand I had done with my right hand. However, all was not good. Though I had "balanced" the opening of the drawer with my left hand with the same action with my right hand, there was now a sequence that needed to be counterbalanced: *open and close dresser drawer with left hand and then open and close the dresser drawer with right hand.* Now, to counter this sequence, I would need to do the following: *open and close the dresser drawer first with my right hand and then open and close the dresser drawer with my left hand.* Here is the only problem: *Though I had balanced the left-right sequence with a right-left sequence, there now existed a left-right-right-left sequence of four that had to be counterbalanced.* The multiplication of sequences would have continued *ad infinitum* if it were not for the limitations of my memory and the fear of being caught.

And to make matters worse, think about how many times a day you have to touch different objects. Now imagine that each time you do so, you have to stop to perform another behavior with the opposite hand to regain a sense of equilibrium. And then try to counter the sequence. It was impossible to keep up. This perfect sense of balance was always one sequence away from my grasp.

Once again, I was losing heart. I was falling short. I could not meet the standard.

* * * * * * *

Every breath seemed tinged with condemnation. Every attempt at restoring balance remained incomplete. Every attempt at prayer fell short. Nothing was ever good enough. I was a failure. It did not matter how hard I tried. The brokenness was so thorough that an intervention was needed. Someone or something from the *outside* would have to interject something into the equation. Left to myself, I was spiraling downward.

43

DAYBREAK

*"The people walking in darkness
have seen a great light; and those
living in the land of deep darkness a
light has dawned."*[43]

Daybreak is that time of day when the sun first appears. The full light and warmth that the sun provides is still hours away. Yet, this "breaking" of the darkness is enough to reassure us that midday is fast approaching when the sun will shine forth in all of its glory.

My *daybreak* moment came in high school while still living under my parent's roof. One night, I was lying on my back in my room about to go to sleep. As I lay there, I began to pray to the Lord. After saying what was on my heart, I did not feel that my prayer was adequate. I always felt this way. Somehow, the words did not come out of my mouth in a perfect manner. So, as usual, I repeated my prayer. Once again, the prayer did not feel good enough. I prayed the exact same prayer again. Over and over again, I continued. I hated prayer. It seemed nothing more than an elaborate, tense collection of repetitions that produced death rather than life.

---

[43] Isaiah 9:2

However, on this particular night, everything would change. Light was about to break through. As I lay on my bed repeating my prayers that night, I did not realize that because of the intense frustration I was feeling, I was getting louder and louder and louder.

The house my family was living in was two-story. My room was upstairs on one end of the hallway, my brother's room was in the middle, and my sister's room was on the other end. I did not know it, but my mom was in my sister's bedroom on the other end of the hallway saying goodnight. All of a sudden, my mom knocked on my door and, in a soft, sweet voice that only a mom can truly pull off. She said, "B.J." in a sort of questioning tone. She opened the door and I immediately asked, "Can you turn the light on?" Though an innocent question, mom later reminded me of this part of the story. You could say that, though I was referring to the physical lights at that moment, the question represented the deeper cry that was burning in my spirit. I needed someone, somehow, to shed some light.

I remember her asking something along the lines of, "Are you okay?" She told me that she heard me from the other end of the hallway. I had no idea that the volume of my prayers had risen to that level.

At first, I was extremely nervous and afraid. My secret had been uncovered. I felt so exposed, so afraid. What would my mom think of me? Who would she tell? Would she think I was as stupid and dumb as I believed I was for these insane struggles? Yet, some other voice in my heart whispered that this, with all of its risks, could be my moment. I did not have the heart to share my struggle. I was too ashamed. If I was going to ever get the help I so desperately needed, God would have no choice but to violate His gentlemanly nature, strip my fig leaves, and leave me naked. This is what He did. It was up to me now to respond. I could lie to my mom and remain hidden, or I could let my fig leaves fall to the ground. I chose to bare my soul. To this day, it may still be the greatest risk of faith I have ever taken.

And then the *unthinkable* happened.

After I had explained what I was doing, my mom sat down on my bed and told me that earlier that week, the Lord had prepared her for this moment. I had no idea what she was talking about. She had watched *Oprah* and the entire show revolved around people suffering from something labeled *Obsessive-Compulsive Disorder*. Think about it. Two to three days before she would "just so happen" to overhear me repeating myself, she watches a show that was dedicated to informing people about this illness. God primed her mind, prepared her heart, and gave her what she would need to make sure she did not dismiss my struggle as insignificant or stupid. If she would have, such a response would have made matters even worse.

God had gone before me. David wrote, "I have set the Lord always before me." I do not remember setting the Lord in front of me, but, praise God, He does not mind taking the initiative. He knew what I needed. He knew that I was nothing more than fancy dust.[44]

Do you see His sovereignty? Do you see the tapestry He was intricately weaving on my behalf? Do you see the detail in His work?

Having never told another human being of my experience, my mom was sitting on the edge of my bed explaining to me the nature of my illness. Did you catch that? I did not say that I was attempting to help her understand. She was putting words to my pain. She was explaining the nature of this illness to me though I was the one who was suffering. There are no words for the relief and hope that was washing over and flooding my heart.

Someone understood.

Someone could now help shoulder my burden.

Someone finally *knew* me and *still* loved me.

Someone was now in my corner and willing to help me stand and fight back.

_____

[44] Psalms 103:14 NKJV

47

This conversation led to many more conversations as well as material (articles and books) that my mom would get for us to study. One thing that deeply impacted my life was that she did not just hand this material to me, but she read it also. She was just as committed as I was to reading, learning, and understanding this illness. She stepped into my darkness with light. I cannot put into words how much love and hope entered my heart for the simple reason that, not only was I no longer alone, but even more importantly, the person by my side was committed to understanding my struggle so she could be there for me in a more effective way.

She hit the light switch. She turned the light on for me.

Daybreak.

God had initiated my journey to freedom.

A THIRD-FLOOR ENCOUNTER

"He brought them out of darkness
and the shadow of death,
and broke their chains in pieces."[45]

I attended Kansas Wesleyan University in Salina, Kansas, where I played basketball in my second semester of college. I had transferred to this college because they offered me a partial scholarship to play. As is common, I shared a room on the third floor in a dormitory on campus. My roommate's family, unlike mine, lived close enough that on the weekends he would sometimes go home. My family lived in Texas, so going home was not an option. Therefore, I had quite a bit of time to myself in that room. This made it easy for me to continue a spiritual practice that I had committed to early in my life. Since age 13, I would get up every morning to read my Bible and pray for a few minutes before leaving for school. As time went on, the amount of time I spent with the Lord grew. God is not afraid of small beginnings.

In the past, my time with the Lord looked different depending on the day. Some days I would spend most of my time reading and praying God's Word. Other days I might turn on worship music and get

---

[45] Psalms 107:14 NKJV

lost in singing songs to Jesus.[46] On this particular occasion, I had done just that. On the third floor of that insignificant little room, David Ruis' vineyard song "Break Dividing Walls" began playing. Suddenly, my physical body felt really weak. Due to the physical weakness, coupled with a desire to humble myself, I knelt. I then remember distinctly feeling too weak to kneel, so I then proceeded to lie face down on the floor. This is probably the closest I have ever come to experiencing what charismatic Christians label "being slain in the Spirit." This was a holy, *burning bush* sort of moment. There are a handful of these moments that God has in store for each person. This was one of mine. I can still visualize the exact place I was lying on the floor, facing south, in that third floor room. Here is my journal entry later that day, March 17th, 1998:

---

[46] These days, I do not vary too much. I actually prefer to spend time with the Lord without music. I begin with a Psalm. I would go more into detail, but I present in detail what my time with the Lord looks like in the morning in another one of my books, *The Word As a Vehicle*.

My God,

What a precious day. I have full faith that this is the day, I have been delivered, you have given me freedom, and I rejoice. As I jumped and danced, you filled me with an overwhelming sense of joy. After I acted a fool for you, I fell to the ground with a sense of heaviness in spirit as tears came forth! I layed on the ground, and the tears still flowed. As they did, I felt freedom. I believe this is the day you chose, March 17, 1998, to give me rest, complete rest from the demonic spirits of OCD and "religious" spirits. My head does not hurt, my mind does not ache. I weep now at the trouble these things have inflicted. These tears are my way of releasing the pain of my past of struggling with these things, and they are at the same time tears of joy, for you have shown me favor today, and you have given me a peace of mind I have cried out for for years. Why today? I know not, but what joy I have. Lately, the devil has attacked me so hard my head has hurt as I have been continually trying to keep evil thoughts out of my mind. I have always done what I can to keep from entertaining them, but just trying to fight them, even with your strength, has taken its toll on me. Literally throughout recent days, my mind and head have even hurt, because I was trying so hard to keep bad thoughts out, so that I would only think in a good way. Even though I didn't entertain the bad thoughts, the "religious" spirits had me in a trap of thinking that just because the devil tempted me with them, I had done wrong. NO MORE! Deliverance and Freedom is mine, and I rejoice. My mind feels so clear and at peace and my head no longer hurts. A miracle you have performed, one that I shall be forever grateful

I do not remember exactly how long that encounter with the Lord lasted. Here is what I do remember: *When I got up off the floor, I knew in my spirit that God had set me free from OCD.* When I say, "in my spirit," I am referring to the deepest part of my being. Paul wrote that a person is spirit, soul, and body.[47] It is possible to know something in your spirit that is impossible to know otherwise. Knowledge of this nature is communicated via *revelation,* whereas knowledge that we have in a more ordinary, mental sort of way is a product of *reason.* Christians believe that one can know something via revelation that is impossible to know by reason alone. This distinction between the

---

[47] 1 Thessalonians 5:23

limited knowledge of reason and the limitless knowledge of revelation is best illustrated in Paul's letter to the Ephesians. He writes, "To know the love of Christ which passes knowledge..."[48] There is a knowledge our minds can reach, and then there is a type of knowledge that skips past the mind. It can only be received.

What is the point in writing all of this?

When I rose from the floor that day, there was absolutely no reason in the natural realm to believe that anything had changed. It was a cold, hard floor. I had heard the song before. I had had hundreds of times with the Lord in the past. What was so special about this particular time on this particular day? From a rational standpoint, *nothing.* From a spiritual standpoint, *everything.* In my spirit, I somehow, someway knew that something was different.

Faith entered my heart that day.

When I stood up, I knew I was free. I knew that in that moment, God the Father, by the presence of His Spirit in that room and in my heart,[49] had applied the power that is in the blood of Jesus Christ to my brokenness (i.e. OCD). We make the tragic mistake sometimes of believing that the power of Jesus Christ is only for the forgiveness of sins; and while

---

[48] Ephesians 3:19 NKJV

[49] Galatians 4:6 (the Spirit being our hearts)

this in itself is absolutely wonderful, this is not the complete picture. The power of Jesus Christ is also for our physical bodies, our emotional pain, insecurity, addictions, and all of the other various forms of brokenness that plague humanity as a direct consequence of our fallen nature. God, using His power through the blood of Christ to forgive sin, is only the beginning of the journey, not the destination. God wants Christians to thrive, to be fully alive, to live awakened. Jesus said, "I have come that they may have life, and that they may have it more abundantly." [50] Receiving God's forgiveness through the atoning, sacrificial, substitutionary work of Christ opens the door to everything else that is in His heart to share with you. Walking through the door of Christ[51] gets you inside the house. You have not even yet begun to explore. The fun is just now starting. There are pantries and closets and *Narnia-esque* wardrobes awaiting you.

At this point, you are probably expecting to hear that shortly thereafter, my struggle with OCD ceased. After all, I stood up that day knowing in my spirit that God had set me free.

But there was a problem.

Not only did the OCD not go away, at times it seemed to be getting worse. The struggle

---

[50] John 10:10
[51] John 10:2

intensified. The fight seemed more difficult than ever before.

MY EARLY 20'S

*"I would have lost heart, unless I
had believed that I would see the
goodness of the Lord in the land of
the living."[52]*

God had already done so much. He had poured such
comfort and hope into my heart by intricately
arranging a series of events that brought my mom
into my struggle. Within a few years, the *third-floor
encounter* occurred. However, as I stated at the end
of last chapter, not only did my OCD not disappear,
it at times seemed worse.

As mentioned earlier, I lived terrified of a bad
thought entering my mind. This was the main way
that Obsessive-Compulsive Disorder plagued me in
my early twenties. Fear reigned. I was unable to
light-heartedly dismiss the impure thoughts because
I could not differentiate between being tempted and
actually sinning. Bad thoughts would pop into my
mind, and I would immediately experience horrible
guilt. The following journal entry, dated September
20, 1999, indicates the extent to which
condemnation and shame had dominated my life:

---

[52] Psalms 27:13 NKJV

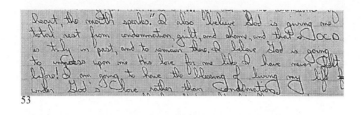

53

The following entry was recorded about a month later on October 11, 1999:

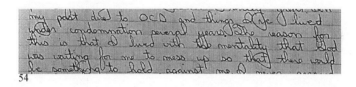

54

The guilt was so intolerable that I would immediately, either in my thoughts or under my breath, confess my sin to God so that I could go on my way. However, it did not work. Again, just like high school, my prayer for God's forgiveness never felt good enough. And when my prayer did not seem good enough, my tendency was to repeat the prayer over and over again until I felt forgiven. The problem was that I never felt forgiven, and so I kept asking, begging, praying. I lived like a beggar, not a son.

When all of this is bouncing around in your head, it is nearly impossible to live in the present tense. You get so caught up in this make-believe world that

---

[53] Technically, I was about a month away from turning 20.

[54] This was recorded a few days before I turned 20.

your heart is not free to step outside of yourself and engage your surroundings. Because of this mental illness, your life becomes all about you. All of your time is channeled inward rather than upward and outward. Dr. Michael Emlet makes this point nicely when he writes, "Recognize the ways in which your obsessions and compulsions keep you from loving those closest to you. Focus on these real sins, instead of the potential sins you have imagined in your mind. Then turn to Jesus Christ in repentance and faith."[55] Now, be careful not to read too much into these words. I do not believe a person sins every time he or she gives into OCD. However, sometimes it can help to face the facts, and the fact is that OCD keeps you wrapped up tightly in your own little world. This grievous reality, I believe, can actually help motivate you to muster up every bit of strength you have to fight!

I was faced with the following dilemma in public settings: *If I do not continually ask God's forgiveness (either in the form of thought-prayers or whispering under my breath) until somehow I feel it, I am stuck with this unbearable guilt. But if I continue, people around me are going to notice that I am staring at the floor, looking off in the distance, or talking to myself.* The thoughts and feelings were

---

[55] "Living with Obsessive-Compulsive Disorder (OCD)," Family Life, accessed November 14, 2014, http://www.familylife.com/articles/topics/life-issues/challenges/mental-and-emotional-issues/living-with-obsessive-compulsive-disorder#.VGYWkohOKrX.

so strong, so overpowering, that the challenge of preventing my inner world from manifesting itself in strange behavior that others might notice was becoming more and more difficult. I had to get away. I needed a place.

So where did I go? *Restrooms.*

I figured out that the closest "sanctuary" in public settings was a bathroom stall. First of all, guys do not talk in a restroom. Second of all, once in a stall, you can lock the door. Third, I knew nobody would peep through the crack to see what I was doing. People would assume I was doing what everyone does in a bathroom stall. Therefore, I would not be questioned. Whether it took me 30 seconds or 5 minutes, I could do what needed to be done in order to quiet my broken conscience.

This actually would have been a pretty good strategy except for one thing: *I was so broken, so ashamed, so "unclean" and "imperfect," that I needed to retreat into a stall on average once every 15-20 minutes.* I was 20 years old at this time, and this, I believe, was probably the worst my symptoms had ever been (and that is no small statement).

I knew that if I made a habit of visiting the restroom every 20 or so minutes, people would start noticing. I had to scratch and claw against my conscience to buy more time between the sanctuary retreats. Yet, this was not always effective. There were times in public I would go to the restroom to find a stall 3-4 times in an hour. I became a master of hiding this behavior as well as giving good explanations. I had to be aware of my surroundings. I might wait till the current group of people walked out of the room so that the new group that hadn't seen my previous trip to the restroom would not think anything of my second or third or fourth visit. To them, they were seeing me go for the first time. Embarrassment avoided. I became a master at juggling. It was complicated. Writing this just now, I had to stop and take a deep breath. I still remember. It was excruciatingly painful and exhausting. My life did not feel like my own and I wanted it back so badly.

Below is a journal entry dated July 25, 2001 (I was 22 years old):

July 25, 2001 TUES.

Yesterday, talking to my mom, and then looking stuff up over the internet, I realized I still have OCD tendencies. It use to be controlling, devestating, it was destroying and killing me. I'm so much better now and yet I can still recognize alot of this behavior in my life. Here is where I recognize it the most. My fear of evil and other perverted thoughts. Sometimes I live in such fear of them that it tenses my body and entraps my mind. I will become timid in engaging with people b/c "what if" my mind goes there. I live in fear of where my mind could go. So many days I will live very tense. All this makes me very anxious, it makes me frustrated, and in the end somewhat depressed and even angry. Medication would and could help me

61

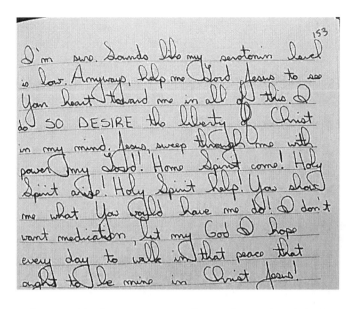

It is an odd phenomenon to know in your spirit that God has declared you free while in the natural realm, what He has declared you free *from* keeps getting worse.

How do I explain that?

How does anyone explain that?

On the one hand, I believed with all of my heart that God had set me free from OCD. However, on the other hand, I could not remember a time when I felt *more* chained. *Prima facie*, this was the ultimate either/or situation. Was I free *or* was I not? Rationality demanded a choice. The *Law of*

Contradiction[56] would not allow for both. There appeared to be an irreconcilable contradiction between the freedom I believed God had granted me and the intensified struggle that I was experiencing. So what gives? Was I free or was I not?

"The law that a proposition (e.g. I am free) cannot be both true and false..." (dictionary.com)

PARADOX

"My people are destroyed for lack of knowledge."[57]

There is a difference between a contradiction and paradox. This lies at the heart of understanding some of the deeper truths of the Christian faith.[58]

Merriam-Webster defines *contradiction* as "a difference or disagreement between two things which means that both cannot be true."[59] Here is an example: *John is a married bachelor*. Both of these facts cannot be true. Either John is married or he is a bachelor. There is no possible way to reconcile a contradiction.

Paradox is defined as "something (such as a situation) that is made up of two opposite things and that seems impossible but is actually true or possible."[60] Here is an example: *I'm a compulsive liar*. So, am I lying when I say that? It would appear that by merely making this assertion I am contradicting myself. I am claiming to always lie while attempting to make a truthful statement about always lying. But, upon closer inspection, I am not

---

[57] Hosea 4:6 NKJV

[58] I am indebted to Bruce Campbell for several of our conversations (more him talking than me) about the nature of *paradox* and the role it plays in the Christian faith.

[59] http://www.merriam-webster.com/dictionary/contradiction

[60] http://www.merriam-webster.com/dictionary/paradox

saying that I lie every single time I speak. What I am actually saying is that more often than not, I lie. It is a regular thing I do. Matter of fact, I am probably lying more often than telling the truth. So, while at first glance it seems the statement, "I'm a compulsive liar," is contradictory, it in fact is not upon closer inspection. A paradox is only contradictory when considered on a surface level. When you look under the hood, the apparent contradiction dissolves.

There are certain truths in the Christian faith that cannot be understood if one does not understand paradox. Put simply, *paradox* plays a significant role in Christianity.

In the previous chapter, I ended with, "Was I free or was I not?" I believed that God had set me free in that third floor dorm room. However, the OCD continued to get worse. Which was it? What I believed God had told me or what I was experiencing? As my senior pastor says, would I believe the facts of my experience or the truth of what God had deposited in my spirit? At a glance, I was asserting two contradictory statements. But upon closer inspection, I was faced with a paradox.

Both statements were true. My OCD was getting worse. However, God had set me free. How can both of these statements be true at the same time for the same person? The answer to this question is one of the great and beautiful mysteries of the Christian faith.

* * * * * * *

Richard Foster writes, "Superficiality is the curse of our age," and, "The desperate need today is not for a greater number of intelligent people, or gifted people, but for deep people."[61] A person who only dabbles in religion will end up walking away for the simple reason that he or she is not prepared to do the work necessary to acquire a deeper understanding. *Work?* You say, "I thought Christianity was a religion of grace? I thought Christ did the work for us?" And you are right. He did. Yet, there is a little more to the picture. He may be providing the food, but for some reason, He still expects you to stop what you are doing, come to the table, sit down, and use your own hand to lift the fork to your mouth. Besides, I doubt a starving individual would dare label the act of picking up a fork "work" if someone was sitting in front of him offering food. He would be glad to do his part. He no doubt would be cognizant of the fact that he was not able to take care of himself, that the work of nourishment was ultimately provided by someone else, but he still had to receive. He still had to chew. He still had to swallow. Let us rid ourselves of this stupid, apathetic image of grace that is crippling Christians everywhere. We have work to do and, though that work may be only a piece of the pie, it

---

[61] Richard Foster, *The Celebration of Discipline* (New York: HarperOne, 1998), 1.

is work nonetheless. If this ruffles your feathers, you might as well pack your bags and go home.

Paul wrote, "...continue to work out your salvation with fear and trembling, for it is God who works in you to will and to act in order to fulfill his good purpose."[62] So...*which is it?* Is God going to do the work or do I need to do it? On the surface, as discussed earlier, this appears to be a clear case of a logical contradiction. But upon closer inspection, we see paradox. There is work for Christians to do in conjunction with the work, the *real* work, that only the Holy Spirit can do. The "work" that I am commanded to do and the work that God is going to do is, at a fundamental level, different from one another. Our work is more of a passive, positional kind. The work of the Holy Spirit is essentially active. He and He alone is the one who has the power to bring about deep and permanent transformation. I cannot do that. What I *can* do is put forth significant effort (i.e. *work*) to place myself in just the right position for Him to complete that work in me.

For example, let's pretend John and Susan's marriage is on the rocks. They are at a standstill and do not know what to do next. Susan says she is done and does not want to work on the marriage. John, on the other hand, wants the marriage to work but is more aware than ever that he does not have the power to change Susan's heart. Then, out of

---

[62] Philippians 2:12-13

nowhere, Susan tells John that, though she does not think there is much hope, she is willing to join him in seeing a counselor if he is still up for it. Now, there is nothing magical about getting into a car, driving a few miles, and sitting in the office of a complete stranger. This by itself will not change anybody's heart. However, nobody would deny that this is a pivotal moment in their marriage. Why? For the simple reason that Susan has agreed, with John, to *change their position*. Before, John had nothing to hold on to for hope. Susan was done, and there was nothing happening that gave John a reason to think, "Well, there is at least a chance that things might turn around." But now, he has hope. He now has a great reason to believe their marriage has a chance. They are getting help. With one decision, they shifted their feet and stood on different ground. A counselor can help them. A third, impartial, neutral voice, might be the only thing that can make the difference. They are now in a position of hope. They did the work. Change is now possible. In this new position, someone can now help them. In our spiritual lives, this "someone" is the Lord. The work of a Christian tends to be more passive in nature, yet it is still crucial in the overall work of Christ.

When you look at Philippians 2:12-13 in this light, the apparent contradiction quickly fades. Paul was saying that each party involved in the relationship had work to do. Granted, God's work is the greater work. He is the one who actually does the transforming. However, you must spend the time and effort and come to the table. It's a dance. *The New American Commentary* states,

> *"Paul presented both the work of God ('works in') and the work of the individual Christian ('work out'). Paul recognized the place of each. Divine initiative called for a human response. While he believed that, ultimately, all of salvation, considered in its broadest scope, depended on God's initiative and power, he never tolerated passive Christianity. Human energy could never accomplish the work of God, yet God did not accomplish his purposes without it. The two [types of work] functioned in perfect harmony..."[63]*

He works. I work. We work together. There is no contradiction here.

* * * * * * *

To return to the issue at hand, the question remains, how was I both "free" and "not free" at the same time?

By *faith*, I was free. God had spoken this into my spirit. He had declared it over me. The chains were snapped. I knew it.

---

[63] Richard R. Melick, *The New American Commentary – Philippians, Colossians, Philemon* (Nashville: Broadman Press, 1991), 111.

In *practice*, I was not free. Matter of fact, the OCD seemed to be getting worse.

Because I had accepted Christ, I received the person of the Holy Spirit. How do I know? This is what I am promised in God's Word. At Pentecost, Peter was preaching to a massive audience. The Bible says the people were "cut to the heart" [64] upon hearing the Gospel. They began to cry out to Peter asking what they needed to do in order to be saved. How should they respond to the message they were hearing? Peter replied, "Repent and be baptized, every one of you, in the name of Jesus Christ for the forgiveness of your sins. And you will receive the gift of the Holy Spirit. The promise is for you and your children and for all who are far off---for all whom the Lord our God will call." [65] When a Christian chooses to trust in Jesus Christ for the forgiveness of sin, God in turn deposits his Holy Spirit in that person.

Why mention this? For the person who has the Holy Spirit, all things are possible. This individual is not limited to his own meager resources. *All* things are possible? Yes. Now, I will admit that sometimes, even though I have faith in Christ, it is hard for me to believe this. Really hard. Sometimes I actually struggle to believe whether God will do anything at all. But I look up, stay in the Word, and try to stay

---

[64] Acts 2:37
[65] Acts 2:38-39

in faith. The Holy Spirit helps. Do you doubt? Do you fear? Do you wonder how long? Me too. And yet, God keeps coming through.

On that third floor in that room, the Holy Spirit had declared in my spirit that I was free. The picture I have always had is this:

> *OCD had built a prison around me. I did not see any way out. I surely did not have the key to my cell door. Someone with greater power would have to intervene. On that day in my dorm room, Christ walked down the hallway and unlocked the prison door. I was free. Although I heard Him say that I was free as He simultaneously turned the key and opened the creaky door, it would be years before I actually found that door. For years, until my freedom was final, I groped around in the thick darkness, desperately trying to find where exactly the door was located. As I felt around, I continually felt bar after bar. I knew I was free. I knew the door was opened. I knew that everything had changed. However, as stated earlier, I had to do some work. My eyes were adjusting. The door was wide open, I just had to find out where it was. Once I did, I would walk free. You might say that I was working hard, searching for the freedom that was already both declared and provided. The hardest work had been done already, the work I had no power to*

accomplish. It was my turn now. I had to walk out.

We are told to walk by faith, not by sight. [66] According to my sight, I was still in prison. According to faith, I had already been set free. *It was just a matter of time before I stepped into the victory that I had already been given.*

You might be wondering, as I have in the past, "Why did God allow this interval of time between the moment He declared me free and the actual manifestation of that freedom in my daily life (i.e. the time I actually starting walking in that freedom)? To be frank, I don't know. I cannot answer this. Sure, it would not require much effort to create a list of potential explanations but, in the end, the list would be nothing more than speculation. I simply do not know why God allowed me to grope around for many more years. It could have been my fault. Maybe it was supposed to be part of my story. Who knows?

But you know what? Who cares! Freedom is freedom. How insane would it be to spend the rest of my life angry at God for letting me grope around for a few more years rather than dancing like a little child in the freedom I have now?

I don't have time to get in bed with the past. The present and the future are far too attractive.

---

[66] 2 Corinthians 5:7

Think about the above prison analogy once again. When Jesus unlocked the prison door and whispered into my heart that I was free, I became certain of it. I had this experience that came furnished with a promise to stand on. What does a promise deliver? *Hope!* A promise delivers hope. A promise can help you trust God. How many times does God declare something that does not come to pass for many, many years?

Sometimes even decades.

Abraham received a promise concerning Isaac at age 75, but Isaac was not born until Abraham was 100. Joseph received his two dreams at age 17. At 30, after immense trial and suffering, the dreams finally came to pass. And then there was David. The prophet Samuel anointed him king as a teenager. After years of running for his life, at age 30, he finally stepped into that role. Moses tended animals in the desert for 40 years before partnering with God to lead one of the great deliverances in Israel's history. Jesus was a "mere" carpenter for the majority of His earthly life. I could continue, but you get the point. God does not seem to be in a hurry. He lost His watch. He doesn't receive notifications. He will allow time to pass that from a human vantage-point feels like an utter waste. All I know is this: *Somehow, in my spirit, I knew that I knew that I knew that God had set me free.* The beauty of this is that, even as my OCD worsened in the natural realm, I had hope. *Against all hope, [I] in hope believed.* [67] Against all hope? Yes. My experience was telling me that I had no reason to hope, that the illness was getting worse. But against this, I, in hope of what God had declared to me on that third floor, enabled me to supernaturally believe that, no matter what my experience was screaming, it was a lie. God cannot lie, and He had said that I was free.

This is the word that carried me forward.

This is the word I stood on when the storm raged.

This is the word that ministered strength to my heart when everything seemed to shout the opposite of what I felt God had declared.

The bottom line is this: *When my heart felt overwhelmed and thoughts and feelings of hopelessness loomed, the word of the Lord supplied me with the power to keep my head up, knowing that my present struggle would not be my future reality.*

The word of the Lord fed my heart the ability to delight in the promise of God that, though delayed, was on its way. Now, do not misunderstand me. The freedom was not on its way. God had declared me free already. What was on its way was the full realization of that freedom in my everyday life. In other words, this promise helped me hang on until I

---

[67] Romans 4:18

saw what I had been already given manifested in my life.

Simply put, I was not yet walking in what I had already been given. But I knew I would stumble into it. I knew it would be realized. I knew that God had already done His work. After years of bondage, disappointment, and heartache, I now had hope. I had something to wait for. The thing I wanted more than anything else had already been promised to me. What would a little more suffering be? Nothing in comparison to the moment that I *now* knew was heading toward me. I was no longer chasing freedom. Jesus had told me that I would have a head-on collision!

The words, "Now faith is being sure of what we hope for and certain of what we do not see,"[68] now made sense to me. My faith in what God had said filled the gap in my heart until the reality of the promise came to pass. Faith is not for faith's sake. That would be totally empty. What is faith for? Reality! Faith is to stand in the gap for that which has not yet arrived until what is being "faithed" appears.

Isaiah once wrote that the coming Christ would fulfill the following: *"The Spirit of the Lord GOD is upon Me, because the LORD has anointed Me to preach good tidings to the poor; He has sent Me to heal the brokenhearted, To proclaim liberty to the*

---

[68] Hebrews 11:1

captives, and the opening of the prison to those who are bound."[69]

Wow! Did you read that? What appropriate language. *The opening of the prison to those who are bound.* In my life, He kept his Word. God is that good. He did not kill me. He healed me.

---

[69] Isaiah 61:1 NKJV

IN THE MEANTIME

*"Idle hands are the Devil's
workshop."*

The experience on the third floor in Salina, Kansas, occurred when I was 19 years old. I groped around in the prison, trying to find the door Jesus had unlocked, until I was 26. Eight years? Again, I do not claim to understand it all.

So what did I do in the meantime between the promise at 19 and the realization of that promise at 26? I did some work. I did what I could. I developed some coping skills while I waited.

I am currently counseling a young man who suffers from OCD. His is not a mild case. It is serious. We have already begun to see some progress. He is a Christian, and while we wait for his freedom, I am now sharing some of the skills with him that helped me.

One of the most effective treatments for OCD in psychology is *Cognitive Behavioral Therapy (CBT)*. The *International OCD Foundation* reports, "CBT is made up of many different kinds of therapies. The most important therapy in CBT for OCD is called

Exposure and Response Prevention (ERP)."[70] The basic idea is to go to the root and stare the problem in the face. One article reads,

> *"The 'Exposure' in ERP refers to confronting the thoughts, images, objects, and situations that make a person with OCD anxious. The 'Response Prevention' in ERP refers to making a choice not to do a compulsive behavior after coming into contact with the things that make a person with OCD anxious. This strategy may not sound right to most people. Those with OCD have probably confronted their obsessions many times and tried to stop themselves from doing their compulsive behavior only to see their anxiety skyrocket. With ERP a person has to make the commitment to not give in and do the compulsive behavior until they notice a drop in their anxiety. In fact it is best if the person stays committed to not doing the compulsive behavior at all. The natural drop in anxiety that happens when you stay 'exposed' and 'prevent' the 'response' is called habituation."[71]*

---

[70] "Cognitive Behavior Therapy," International OCD Foundation, accessed October 2, 2014, http://iocdf.org/about-ocd/treatment/cbt/.

[71] International OCD Foundation, "Cognitive Behavior Therapy."

In other words, you are changing your behavior with the intent of ultimately retraining your emotions. *Habituation* is really nothing more than learning new habits. There is such a thing as an emotional habit. These also need resetting.

Though one of my undergraduate degrees is in psychology, I started applying this method in my own life before I ever came across this information. It was more difficult and gut-wrenching than I can put into words. The old saying, "It may get worse before it gets better," was definitely true. This is actually what is so challenging about treatment. We as humans are not good at subjecting ourselves to something that produces discomfort. The truth is, sometimes discomfort is the only way to travel from a hopeless point A to a hopeful point B. One must embrace discomfort. William Backus writes, "Discomfort never killed anyone."[72] This is true, but knowing this and acting on it are two different things.

Luckily, I chose to embrace discomfort. It helped significantly. Some days were better than others. But even on the worst days, I had God's promise of a coming freedom upholding my heart. I could fight the *battle* because the Lord had told me that the *war* had already been won. I was free. I just wasn't walking in freedom yet.

---

[72] William Backus, *Telling Yourself the Truth* (Minnesota: Bethany House Publishers, 1980), 22.

What did ERP look like in my life? My prayer life was one of the main ways I implemented this technique. What I found was that OCD mainly disrupted my prayers when I was confessing sin. I would pray, then pray again, and keep repeating myself until I finally said everything in a perfect way so that I could "feel" forgiven. Living by your feelings in any area of life is foolish and dangerous. You are setting yourself up for confusion and failure. This area was no exception.

So, I began to "bind" myself with a promise. I would pray, "God, I promise on Your name, Your holy name, that what I am about to say I will only say once more." Why would I do this? Well, I intuitively knew I needed something more powerful than my anxiety to keep me from repeating the compulsory behavior aimed at alleviating the anxiety. Because of my faith, I knew that to make a promise to God and break it was a serious deal. The idea of not keeping a promise to God was so disdainful to me that I would pray, confess, repent, and then leave it alone. I had to trust that it was good enough, because, if I did not, my options were twofold: (1) break my promise and repeat, or (2) be miserable the rest of the day. I began, little by little, to actually receive God's forgiveness in my heart. I wanted peace. I wanted joy. God had promised these things to every Christian and I wanted what was rightfully mine (i.e. inheritance).

Some days, I went back on my promise. I would undo the promise, make the promise again, and then pray one more time. On these days, I would not experience much relief. I was still repeating myself. As a matter of fact, when the "binding" was not working so well, all it did was further complicate the process.

Though I have broken many promises to the Lord, along the way I had to realize that I was very flawed and this was the best I could do until His promised freedom was activated. I was trying to give myself a little bit of grace. Sometimes it worked; sometimes it didn't. At least I was trying. At least I was not throwing in the towel.

If I remember correctly, I did apply this "binding" strategy in other areas as well. I would tell God, "I promise You that I, upon flipping this switch one more time, will not do it again for the next hour." Why the next hour? Because I knew that I was about to leave for the day, so by setting this time limit I would not be able to hit the switch again until I returned later that day. Life seemed to be a mental circus at times. But again, I was doing what I could to cope while waiting for my promise.

I could walk you through each and every specific example, but this should suffice. I believed that it was such a big deal to break a promise to God that for the most part, by promising to Him that I would not do something again, I was effectively using Him to enact ERP in my personal life. The *International OCD Foundation* reports, "For the people who benefit from CBT, they usually see their OCD

81

symptoms reduced by 60-80%."[73] In my case, I am not sure my percentage was quite so high, but my "spiritual" version of ERP definitely helped.

But didn't Jesus say,

> *"Again you have heard that it was said to those of old, 'You shall not swear falsely, but shall perform your oaths to the Lord.' [34] But I say to you, do not swear at all: neither by heaven, for it is God's throne; [35] nor by the earth, for it is His footstool; nor by Jerusalem, for it is the city of the great King. [36] Nor shall you swear by your head, because you cannot make one hair white or black. [37] But let your 'Yes' be 'Yes,' and your 'No,' 'No.' For whatever is more than these is from the evil one."[74]*

Yes, He did. So how could I use *promises* and *swears* to keep OCD at bay without sinning? To be honest, I am not sure. Maybe I was sinning. But there just came a point when I did not know what else to do. It was between the Lord and me. I believe that He was grieving over my brokenness and giving me grace as I struggled in my blood.[75] I do not intend to minimize sin. After all, sin required

---

[73] International OCD Foundation, "Cognitive Behavior Therapy."

[74] Matthew 5:33-37 NKJV

[75] This "struggling in my blood" language is from Ezekiel 16:6.

the slaughter of God's Son. That being said, God saw my heart. The only thing I was trying to do was inch closer to the freedom He had promised. And, I was also just trying to get through the day.

If you are struggling with OCD, do your best to implement ERP. It does not matter how small you start, just start! Find it within yourself to resist the urge to always give in to the compulsory behaviors that typically reduce the anxiety. I know what you are thinking: *Yeah, if only it was that easy.* Remember, I am writing to you as someone who has also suffered from this illness. There just comes a point where you have to push back.

It gets worse before it gets better. But it does get better...*eventually.*

For a time period, when you first start to deny the urges you have for so long given into, your anxiety will seem almost unbearable. But over time, if you are somewhat consistent, the level of anxiety will transition from *unbearable* to *uncomfortable*. Then, the anxiety will transition from *uncomfortable* to *tolerable*. Your behavior is the gateway to either reinforcing or retraining your emotions. It is a painful process, no doubt. However, this can significantly reduce your misery until total freedom comes. There is hope, but as I have counseled the young man recently, "Prepare yourself. You are in for the fight of a lifetime."

In all honesty, *Exposure and Response Prevention* was only partially successful. It was helpful in helping me function on a daily basis. Granted, there were days it did not seem to help. This is definitely *not* the final solution. Yet in the short term, it can be quite beneficial. It can buy you time and offer you a little relief.

Though I am not going to spend much time on this, it is important for family members to realize that they play a pivotal role in the ERP process. You must be supportive and at the same time be willing to challenge the individual to push back. When the person fails, there will be times to give grace and encouragement. However, there will also be times when that person needs you to get in his face and remind him (or her) of what life is going to look like down the road if something does not change. Like any relationship, you must know when to extend a tender kind of love and when to give tough love.[76] You will need the Holy Spirit. He can help you discern.

And to the person with OCD, you must give certain family members that you trust (i.e. you are 100% confident that they have your best interest at heart) total access to speak into your life. It will be worth it. Also, every time they speak, you will be reminded that you are not alone anymore in your

---

[76] For Christians, these two kinds of love is best modeled in Christ Himself. He is described in the Bible as both the *lion* and the *lamb*.

struggle. In reference to a study done by Meyers in 1966, Davison and Neale write, "Generalization of the treatment [ERP] to the home required the involvement of family members."[77] You cannot do this alone. If you want freedom, you must give total access to someone who is willing walk beside you.

We all need each other. You are not going far alone. Let people in. And if you are the person being invited in, walk in love and decide now that you will do all that is in your power to be a source of life and hope as opposed to death and discouragement. You will not fully understand, but you don't have to. Just love! Do the best you can. Ask questions. Be a pillar. Be a fountain.

So in the meantime, before your freedom breaks through, do what you can. Push back. Implement ERP. Dare to believe that things can change. Your life can be different. And if you are smart, realize that you need God now more than ever before. Let Him in. Let others in. At this point, what do you have to lose? And remember, as you step out on the water, your anxiety will skyrocket. It will get worse before it gets better. Discomfort is your gateway. Your companion. You cannot get *there* from *here* without it.

---

[77] Davison and Neale. *Abnormal Psychology*. 150.

GRACE WORKS

*"He also brought me out into a
broad place;
He delivered me because He
delighted in me. "*[78]

You never know what God has waiting for you
around the corner. Sometimes you round the corner
only to find, well, nothing in particular. It is just
another day.

And then there is the corner that *seems* just like
every other corner, but is not. This one is different.
This corner was prepared for you. God has a special
package waiting for you. You did not see it coming.
The sun looks different, the temperature has
changed, and you sense that you have stumbled into
a divine appointment.

I rounded one of these corners in my life at age 26.
It would prove to be the last leg on my road to
freedom. I would round what seemed like *just*
another corner to find that Jesus was waiting for me.
God was about to finish what He had started when I
was a teenager. My journey to freedom that had
begun with my wonderful momma walking down
the hallway was coming to a close. Little did I know
that the next corner I was about to round was one of

---

[78] Psalms 18:19 NKJV

those corners that would change the streets I walk on from that point forward. I had no idea that this mental and emotional cripple was *finally* about to dance.

I had finished my undergraduate work in Kansas City and was once again living in my hometown. The youth pastor at my dad's church had stepped down. My dad prayerfully extended the invitation to come serve as the youth pastor at Grace Fellowship Ministries. After a few weeks of prayer, I accepted. Jesus was calling me to partner with my earthly dad in order to serve my other Dad.

It was a tough time in the life of the church, but a time I will never forget. Regarding OCD, I was doing okay. I was not free, but I was functioning decently. However, after so many years of performing in my prayer life due to the OCD, I still never felt good enough for God. I never felt like He liked me. Sure, as a pastor, I spent a significant amount of time telling people of God's wonderful and delightful grace. I would then walk away and say to myself, "You don't even believe it." I did, but only in my head, not my heart. One thinker said, "The greatest distance in the world between two points is the 18 inches between a person's mind and heart." Paul drew a clear distinction between these two kinds of knowing in Ephesians when he wrote, "...to know the love of Christ which passes knowledge; that you may be filled with all the fullness of God."[79] How can you "know" something that passes *knowledge*? You can't, unless there are two different kinds of knowledge. Paul was telling us that there is a knowledge of the heart that is far greater, far more valuable, far more penetrating, than head knowledge. I only possessed head knowledge of God's love. In my heart, I knew that I did not know God's love. I also knew that I had not truly received God's forgiveness in a way that it was touching the emotional part of my nature. I needed help. Intervention. And once again, God would not disappoint. He sits on the edge of His throne, tapping His feet, willing and waiting to crash our party. This is not a game to Him. He laughs and He cries. He dances and He grieves. His words at any moment might be poetry or a song of lament. If you look into His eyes, there is always a glimmer of hope. He is good. He is powerful. And He is ready to get His hands dirty. He specializes in the nitty-gritty. He rushes to what others run away from.

One day, while talking with my dad, he mentioned a series by Clark Witten about grace. I desperately wanted to enjoy God, and, I believed that the Scriptures supported this desire.

I wanted to know what it was like to wake up and feel God's pleasure in my heart.

---

[79] Ephesians 3:19 NKJV

I wanted to know what it was like to be able to immediately drink in God's delightful forgiveness even after I had sinned.

I wanted to stop taking myself so seriously.

I wanted to live outside of my head.

I wanted to know what it was like to spend time with the Lord because I loved Him (as opposed to merely trying to avoid feelings of guilty and condemnation when I didn't).

In good *Kantian* fashion, I had done my best to keep my duty. I was the committed older brother in the story of the *Prodigal Son*.[80] However, I was miserable. Authors Tim Clinton and Pat Springle write, "The intensity of our delight in God is a measuring stick of our grasp of his grace."[81] What I felt in my heart about God was not the person the Bible described. The two were not synced, and I (as well as others) was paying the price.

And then, Daddy God dropped a bread crumb.[82] In the sermon series I was listening to, Clark mentioned a book by Dudley Hall titled "Grace Works." I did not think too much of it. I made a

---

[80] Luke 15:11-32

[81] Tim Clinton and Pat Springle, *Break Through: When to Give In, How to Push Back* (Brentwood: Worthy Publishing, 2012), Kindle.

[82] From the story *Hansel and Gretel*

mental note of the book and then continued to listen. What happened next still produces worship in my heart.

A couple of weeks later, I was walking around in a Christian bookstore at a church in Dallas. I was stopped dead in my tracks when all of a sudden there it was—*Grace Works*. This was the book Clark Witten had mentioned. I am no *spiritual* rocket scientist, but I can put two-and-two together. God was repeating Himself. He had led me to this book through a strategic series of events. Faith grew in my heart that He would not have gone to all of this intricate trouble unless He had chosen this book to bring about something special in my life. I immediately bought it!

God knew three things that I did not know. First, He knew that this was the book He was going to use to do a great work of grace in my life. Second, He knew that within a couple of weeks I would be two hours away in a bookstore that had this book in stock. But, as with any book store, there are a ton of books to pick from. So, He made sure to lead me to this audio series that just so happened to mention this book so that a couple of weeks later, when I saw it, it would stand out. And third, God knew that this book, though it appeared to have nothing to do with OCD, was the key to *my* freedom. The Holy Spirit could see the roots.

Each person is a tree. Most problems people want to talk about are mere tree branches stemming from some deeper root issue. Heal the roots and the entire tree will be healthy. This is what the Holy Spirit was doing in my life. He skipped past the cognitive and behavioral surface issues and got to the root. One of the names that Jesus was given by Isaiah some 700 years before He was born was *Wonderful Counselor.* Christ is the ultimate psychologist. David wrote,

> *You have searched me, Lord, and you know me. You know when I sit and when I rise; you perceive my thoughts from afar. You discern my going out and my lying down; you are familiar with all of my ways. Before a word is on my tongue you, Lord, know it completely.*[83]

He knows us unlike any other. You may be focusing on the superficial issues that *seem* like the problem, but He will, if you are willing, show you the root and deal with the problem. A.W. Tozer writes, "The man who comes to a right belief about God is relieved of ten thousand temporal problems."[84] He is a *root* kind of God. As the Psalmist writes, "He heals the brokenhearted and binds up their wounds."[85] Superficialities bore Him. He is in the business of complete restoration.

---

[83] Psalms 139:1-4
[84] A.W. Tozer, *The Knowledge of the Holy* (San Francisco: HarperSanFrancisco, 1961), 2.
[85] Psalms 147:3 NKJV

To this day, I am still amazed at God's work. Do you see the tapestry? The threads? The goodness in His heart? From my dad to the audio series to the book, God had left a breadcrumb trail for me. I found it. In all truth, it found me. It was almost impossible to miss.[86] Just like the ancient Israelites, God was determined to carry me into the promise land. As the writer of Hebrews states, "There remains, then, a Sabbath-rest for the people of God; for anyone who enters God's rest also rests from their works, just as God did from his. Let us, therefore, make every effort to enter that rest..."[87] A person's *promise land* always delivers the internal mental, emotional, and spiritual rest that is craved. To put it simply, there is no better place to be than in the presence of the Lord and at the center of what He has for you. His presence and His will absolutely include your total freedom. He can get you there. He *will* get you there.

David had it right when he wrote, "Your mercy, O Lord, is in the heavens; Your faithfulness reaches to the clouds."[88]

* * * * * * *

I have told many people that, from the time I started the book to the time I finished, I was a different

---

[86] Which is also part of God's grace. He is not playing games with us. He does not tease.
[87] Hebrews 4:9-11a NKJV
[88] Psalms 36:5 NKJV

person. There are many good books (as well as bad ones). I love to read. I gain information, wisdom, insight, as well as pleasure from books. But this book was different. God breathed through this book into my spirit, soul, and body. The Holy Spirit transformed me through *Grace Works*. Every Jesus follower needs this book right beside their Bible.[89]

I finished reading *Grace Works* 10 years ago. I have NEVER again struggled with whether or not God loves me and delights in me. Deep in my heart, I both know and enjoy God's love in the most personal way. My heart is so, so free. I do not have to walk around every day reciting passages about God's love in an effort to deterministically convince myself that He is not against me. The truth, wonder, and pleasure of His love is now like a fountain that springs up every day within my spirit and heart. I wake up and know He likes me. Experiencing the joy and delight of His love is not something I have to manufacture anymore. I do not have to work my way into it. It is as if it is happening *to* me. Someone else is driving, pouring, lavishing, spilling. There is nothing I have to do to conjure it up. I am the object of God's love. The peace, joy, and freedom His love produces are now the *default* position of my heart. The Bible says, "For the

---

[89] Brennan Manning's three books, *The Ragamuffin Gospel, Ruthless Trust,* and *All Is Grace* are also great books about grace. However, I emphasize *Grace Works* for the simple reason that it is the particular book God used powerfully in my personal journey.

kingdom of God is not a matter of eating and drinking, but of righteousness, peace, and joy in the Holy Spirit."[90] Jesus was establishing His kingdom in my life. Now, I am only conscious of His love. I cannot help it. Anything I do, whether reading the Scripture or serving someone, is merely to express His love rather than try to earn it. He has captured my heart. He led my *captivity* captive.[91]

The question now remains, "How was this event the last leg in my journey to freedom from OCD?" After all, this book was in no way directed toward people who are mentally ill. The words "obsessive" and "compulsive" never appear in the book. But as I stated earlier, the Holy Spirit had fixed His sights on the root of my illness. I had no idea what was about to happen. I just thought my relationship with God was going to improve.

Earlier in the book, I presented one-by-one all of the specific ways that OCD manifested itself in my life. After each one in particular, I wrote, "I was losing heart. I was falling short. I could not meet the standard." Every compulsory behavior I gave into to eliminate the obsession-produced anxiety directly stemmed from this incessant, gnawing feeling in my gut that nothing I did was good enough. No matter how hard I tried, there was some elusive standard that was always a little too high. I was not capable

---

[90] Romans 14:17

[91] "You have ascended on high, you have led captivity captive." Psalms 68:18 NKJV

of performing an activity, any activity, perfect enough. My emotions never let me off the hook and Satan was doing a mighty fine job of lying to me through my emotions. Whether it was flipping a switch and a bad word entering my mind, trying to regain a sense of equilibrium through a complex balancing act, or attempting to say the "just right" prayer, I always fell short. I could not measure up. This realization tortured and abused my every moment.

I needed a personal revelation of God's grace. Clinton and Springle said it perfectly when they wrote, "The intensity of our delight in God is a measuring stick of our grasp of his grace."[92] This is what was missing. I was enslaved to this notion that if I somehow did not satisfy this elusive, *Platonic*[93] ideal of perfection in *every* single area of my life, I failed. In other words, performance, not delight, was what I believed made God tick. God could not smile at me. God could not be pleased with me. God did not want anything to do with me.

I was wrong.

---

[92] Clinton and Springle, *Breaking Through: When to Give In, How to Push Back*, Kindle.

[93] In Plato's *Allegory of the Cave*, there are two worlds, the *World of Appearance* and the *World of Forms*. Though immaterial, the *World of Forms* is the highest, truest realm of reality from which all things in the *World of Appearance* participate in order to gain whatever level of reality the object possesses. The *Forms* are perfect.

Now, do not misunderstand me; perfection is required in order to be in right standing with God, and this is why somebody perfect (i.e. Jesus) had to come take my place on that old rugged cross. His death became my death because the law had to be kept perfectly in order for me to walk with God. When a person says yes to Christ, his sin is imputed to Christ and the perfection of Christ (i.e. righteousness) is imputed to him. All is made right. But notice, this right-standing with God is accomplished through Christ's performance and through His performance alone. Paul wrote, "For it is by grace you have been saved, through faith— and this is not from yourselves, it is the gift of God—not by works, so that no one can boast." One cannot do enough good deeds to earn right-standing with God. In his letter to the church in Colosse, Paul wrote, "He forgave us all our sins, having canceled the charge of our legal indebtedness, which stood against us and condemned us; he has taken it away, nailing it to the cross." Only Christ could accomplish this. A sinful person cannot do away with his own sins. Someone perfect had to take our place. Christ did. By faith, not works, is one made perfect in the eyes of God.

But this is not the perfection I am referring to. I knew that I had to trust Christ for my salvation. The problem was that I was refusing to trust Christ for everything else. In other words, Christ saved me, but now it was my job to sanctify myself. He got things started, but now it was up to me to finish. What a brutal, unforgiving weight.

I needed to come to the place where I realized that the Lord was looking at my heart. God once instructed the prophet Samuel, "Do not look at his appearance or at his physical stature, because I have refused him. For the LORD does not see as man sees; for man looks at the outward appearance, but the LORD looks at the heart."[94] The realization that I had to come to was that my sanctification (i.e. the working out of my salvation) required just as much of God as salvation. We are dependent on the Lord for both. The beginning, the process, and the end belongs to the Lord. This was one of the main reasons that Paul had to write a letter to the church in Galatia. He wrote,

> *"O foolish Galatians! Who has bewitched you that you should not obey the truth, before whose eyes Jesus Christ was clearly portrayed among you as crucified? [2] This only I want to learn from you: Did you receive the Spirit by the works of the law, or by the hearing of faith? [3] Are you so foolish? Having begun in the Spirit, are you now being made perfect by the flesh?"[95]*

The Lord showed me that as long as I am doing my best, giving all of my heart, that it was good enough for Him. Yes, He wants us to grow. He expects us over time, in partnership with Him, to look more

---

[94] 1 Samuel 16:7 NKJV
[95] Galatians 3:1-3 NKJV

and more like Christ. As Brennan Manning writes, "To be like Christ is to be a Christian."[96] That being said, all I can do in the present tense is open my heart to Him and do the best with what He has given me in that moment. That pleases Him. He is not hard to please.

As I read the book, the Holy Spirit completely reprogrammed my thinking. I finished knowing something deep in my heart (and not just in my head): *that God loved me, cared deeply for me, and was actually delighted in my efforts to bring Him pleasure, even when I failed.*

The bottom line is this: *My OCD was rooted in Perfectionism and, as God dealt with that, the OCD lost its power.* There was no more wood for the fire. No more fuel. It had no choice but to die.

Merriam-Webster defines *Perfectionism* as "a disposition to regard anything short of perfection as unacceptable."[97] Add to this a mistaken image of God as a *Tyrant Accountant* and what you have is the worst form of Perfectionism - *the spiritual kind.* As horrible as it is, Perfectionism becomes ten times worse when coupled with a task-oriented, *to-do list* interpretation of Christianity. All potential for *life* is suffocated. Over time, you become numb. *Numbness* is the psyche's way of discharging some

---

[96] Brennan Manning, *Ruthless Trust: The Ragamuffin's Path to God* (San Francisco: HarperSanFrancisco, 2000), 177.
[97] http://www.merriam-webster.com/dictionary/perfectionism

of the momentary emotional weight of guilt, condemnation, anger, disgust, and self-hatred. You have to catch your breath. And, because of this God who accepts nothing but perfection, you have to get as far away as possible. Sure, you may continue to breathe, but that is all.

The University of Illinois' counseling center reports,

> *"Perfectionism refers to a set of self-defeating thoughts and behaviors aimed at reaching excessively high unrealistic goals. Perfectionism is often mistakenly seen in our society as desirable or even necessary for success. However, recent studies have shown that perfectionistic attitudes actually interfere with success. The desire to be perfect can both rob you of a sense of personal satisfaction and cause you to fail to achieve as much as people who have more realistic strivings."*[98]

If perfection is the only tolerable standard (both to God and yourself), then you have two options after completing a task imperfectly. You can either quit trying and accept failure or keep trying until you get it right. But, you can't get it right. Perfection is brutal, unkind, unforgiving. It will not negotiate. It

---

[98] "Perfectionism," Counseling Center at the University of Illinois Urbana-Champaign, accessed November 28, 2014, http://www.counselingcenter.illinois.edu/self-help-brochures/academic-difficulties/perfectionism/.

beats you. It looks you in the eye every time you attempt something to whisper again and again, "You do not have what it takes. You are a failure. You are not good enough." Someone once told Dudley Hall that Christians are miserable because "they are suffering from hardening of the 'oughteries.' They never feel they have done as much as they ought to have done."[99] I would add that this is not only in reference to the quantity of one's work, but also the quality. All falls short. All is inadequate. All is failure when juxtaposed to perfection.

This is actually where the good news begins. Paul wrote, "For all have sinned and fall short of the glory of God."[100] Daddy knew He would have to remedy the sin-situation if it was going to be fixed. And He did, through Christ. Nothing was left undone. All you have to do is call on the name of the Lord with all of your heart.[101]

And once you have, everything changes. You become God's child.[102] You become God's friend.[103] And with the standard of perfection already legally satisfied on your behalf via Christ, you are free to swim around in the love of God. All offenses have

[99] Dudley Hall, *Grace Works* (Ann Arbor: Servant Publications, 1992), 19.
[100] Romans 3:23 NKJV
[101] Romans 10:13
[102] John 1:12
[103] John 15:15

been erased between you and Daddy. Because Christ became perfection for us, all that God looks for now is *heart.* Are you trying? Are you doing your best? Are you showing up? Are you learning? Are you falling on Him when you sin? Are you trusting and delighting in Him the moment after you sin? Christ becomes your answer for everything. He became mine, and this suffocated OCD in my life.

God's *grace* set me free. Merriam-Webster defines *grace* as, "unmerited divine assistance given humans for their regeneration or sanctification."[104] Grace is a gift. It can only be received. The harder you work for it, the further away it is. If you want a religion of works, go elsewhere. Christianity is for the sick people, the incapables, and the have-nots. Sure, rich people are welcome. Capable people are welcome. But at the end of the day, only the *poor in spirit* get in. You must dip low and humble yourself. There is no other way. The best you have will stink up the room. All is grace. God shows His children favor and offers His wonderful assistance because He loves. Period.

After I caught a glimpse of God's grace, notice how my answers changed to some of the challenges OCD presented to me. This will help you see how understanding grace for the first time in my life was the final leg of my journey to freedom.

* * * * * * *

---

[104] http://www.merriam-webster.com/dictionary/grace

Let us begin with prayer. I always repeated my prayers because they never felt perfect. I would always answer no to the self-imposed question, "Did I pray the right way?" But now, with an understanding of grace, my answer changed. Rather than answer the question, "Did I pray the right way?" with either a yes or no, I answered, "Christ."

Did I pray the right way? *Christ.*

Huh? Because of the work of Christ, the question was no longer, "Did I pray perfectly?" Rather, the question became, "Did I pray from and with my heart?" And even this question seems a little intimidating. The question might just be, "Did you give your best shot at praying from your heart?" God's grace, His unearned favor, freed me to take my eyes off of my performance and put them on Him, where they needed to be in the first place. Besides, focusing on your own shortcomings is just another form of self-centeredness. Dudley Hall writes, "The real prisoners in life are those whose focus is on themselves."[105]

When I pray, I now look at Jesus. I trust in Jesus. I laugh at my lack of perfection because of the power of Jesus to make everything acceptable to Daddy. When I do not know how to pray or feel like I used the wrong words, it does not matter. He loves the movements of my heart toward Him. He knows

---

[105] Dudley Hall, *Grace Works*, 87.

what I am trying to say before I say it. I am released from the inner demand to communicate perfectly. Am I praying to Jesus? Yes. Am I becoming more and more a person of prayer? I think so. Does He already know what is in my heart? Of course.

When this revelation consumed me, I realized that a cuss word entering my mind was not that big of a deal. A prayer that did not come out worded perfectly was completely ok. David wrote, "Before a word is on my tongue you, Lord, know it completely."[106] And it was Jesus who said, "Your Father knows what you need before you ask him." [107] So what is there to be uptight about? *Nothing!* In Christ, I am released from that crazed, anxiety-ridden, fear-based demand to pray in a perfect manner. There is no such thing and even if there were, such an ideal would probably not be attractive. I want relationship. God wants relationship. Any time a person in a relationship feels immense pressure to perform in just the right way to be accepted, there is no chance for intimacy there. Intimacy requires that a person knows the other will love him and accept him in spite of imperfection. This acceptance paves the way for love, and nothing has more power to transform a person than love. In the context of love, genuine change can occur. Nothing can move you closer to perfection than love. How ironic that striving for perfection removes you from experiencing God's

---

[106] Psalms 139:4
[107] Matthew 6:8

love though it is that love that holds more power than anything else to perfect you!

* * * * * *

What about the light switches? *Christ.*

What? You may be thinking, "Ugh, here we go again." But that really is my answer. The only reason I flipped those stupid switches over and over and over was because I was trying to flip the switch in just the right way. I had to do it without a cuss word entering my mind. But now, *grace.* Do I now enjoy flipping a switch without be tormented with cuss words? Absolutely. Of course, after writing this, I am sure this is going to happen several times today. But looking back, all I was trying to do was flip a switch *perfectly.* I believed I was extremely displeasing to God because I was not able to flip a switch with pure thoughts. Again, there was this standard of perfection I could not satisfy no matter how hard I tried.

But God.

Now, I understand that it is absolutely NO BIG DEAL that profane words enter my mind when flipping a switch. Who cares! It is just a thought. Temptation is not the same thing as sin. God is not expecting me to flip switches with a pure mind. He wants me to trust Him. *Christ alone.* I do not have to justify myself. Christ already justified me. He already made me good enough.

104

Let me take it a step further. If I am really honest, I believe God's grace is so deep and so rich that He would have rather I went ahead and cussed and repented while flipping a switch than live in such a grievous fear of Him. At least if I had cussed and repented I might have seen just how good and merciful He was, and that probably would have done more to keep me from sinning in the future than all of my futile, sweaty efforts to attain perfection. Besides, which was worse? Saying a cuss word or not trusting in the atoning work of Christ? Saying a cuss word or not believing that God was for me?[108]

I am afraid to write what I am about to write because "Christians" who do not really desire to please God will take it out of context. But I am going to say it anyway. God is so good, so relationship-focused, so concerned with healing our brokenness, that I believe He would rather us go ahead and sin than live with a tormenting fear of sin that destroys any and all potential for authentic relationship with Him. At some point, you must look upon the cross, see the perfect sacrifice of Christ as *your* death, and kneel with joy even as He bleeds. You have permission to quit trying so hard. He has made you good enough. He bled for you in order to give you unobstructed access to Daddy. No more shenanigans are needed. Relax. God is now a safe place for you.

---

[108] Romans 8:31

* * * * * * *

When I finished *Grace Works*, I understood God's grace in my heart. I knew His grace *personally*. It was not an idea or a mask I was trying to wear. When I finished that book years ago, I was changed. It was not gradual. The Holy Spirit deposited a personal understanding of God's grace in my heart as I read. The work felt completed when I finished. It just happened. And as a result, OCD evaporated. God, in His infinite wisdom, knew that my Obsessive-Compulsive Disorder was rooted in Perfectionism, and by ministering His grace to my mind and heart, I would be free. As crazy as it might seem, OCD was a mere symptom. The root was Perfectionism. He took care of my root problem and the rest of the tree became healthy. Daddy God, in His infinite wisdom and power and compassion, delivered me. It was over. At 26 years of age, I stepped into the freedom He had declared in my spirit many years before.

Jesus Christ can do in you what He did in me. I suspect that this book might give people hope in other areas as well. If you have never felt hopeless, you are only half-human. We all need help. We all need grace. We all need someone from the outside to intervene. Another voice is needed, and Christ waits on the edge of His seat to fill that void.

My journey was long. Please do not get discouraged wherever you are at on your path. Good things take time. If you open your heart to Christ, lay your broken self at the foot of the cross, lean into Daddy's chest, open up to someone you trust, and quit trying so hard, Daddy will help you find your way home. You will be alright. Take Jesus' hand and start your journey. He has gone before you.[109] He has already set into motion strategic encounters and events that will ultimately result in your freedom. And one day, you will be able to share your miraculous Jesus story with someone who desperately needs hope. Get going. You cannot afford to wait.

The Lord bless you and keep you;
The Lord make his face shine on you and be
gracious to you;
The Lord turn his face toward you and give you
peace.[110]

---

[109] Psalms 16:8 NKJV
[110] Numbers 6:24-26

APPENDIX A

IS IT MORALLY WRONG FOR A CHRISTIAN TO TAKE MEDICATION FOR MENTAL ILLNESSES?

In my opinion, no!

My official stance on the matter is that medication is a short-term crutch that can help stabilize a person long enough for that person to get *real* help. By *real* help I mean that of a psychological and, above all, *spiritual* nature. If OCD was nothing more than a biological phenomenon, then medication would completely resolve the issue. But it does not. There are deeper roots. However, some cases are extreme and the individual would not be able to endure any other type of treatment without the medication. Medication buys time. It can create space for a person to go deeper, get to the roots, and deal with OCD at such a level that, eventually, the medication will no longer be necessary.

The following statement by Dr. Emlet puts it best. He writes,

> *Research shows that the brain of someone actively struggling with OCD is functioning differently than the brain of a normal person. And yet, the treatment that has the longest and best track record of*

success in the secular world is not medication, but counseling that specifically targets the obsessive thinking and compulsive behavior (commonly called "cognitive-behavior therapy" or "exposure and response prevention therapy"). Over time, as someone responds differently to his obsession (takes the thought less seriously, gives up the quest to control anxiety, and refrains from carrying out a compulsive behavior), his brain activity patterns may well change back toward normal.

However, if the struggle with OCD is so severe that it significantly disrupts daily life and relationships, then medication may be a helpful treatment, along with counseling. The use of these medications may enable you to more thoughtfully and prayerfully engage in the hard work of counseling. [111]

I believe that a person, especially a Christian, should always keep in clear sight the goal of eventually weaning off of medication. A gradual weaning is absolutely preferred. I also believe this is a decision to be made jointly with your caretaker(s) as well as your doctor. However, if the doctor is of the type that he or she does not believe in God, this could complicate things. You must make sure to have a doctor that shares your same

---

[111] Family Life, "Living With Obsessive-Compulsive Disorder (OCD)."

vision. Medication buys you time while you do the hard work of counseling.

Granted, when you first quit taking medication, you may experience all kinds of emotions. It will probably be difficult and scary at first. But, you can do it. If you really sense you are ready to take the step, share this with your caretaker(s) and doctor. You would be wise to heed Solomon's wisdom. Look at the following three scriptures:

"Where there is no counsel, the people fall. But in the multitude of counselors there is safety."[112]

"Without counsel, plans go awry, but in the multitude of counselors they are established."[113]

"For by wise counsel you will wage your own war, and in a multitude of counselors there is safety."[114]

Do not go alone. Do not make these kind of decisions on your own. That being said, it is important that the people you are listening to trust you to some extent and will take your request to wean off medication seriously.

---

[112] Proverbs 11:14 NKJV
[113] Proverbs 15:22 NKJV
[114] Proverbs 24:6 NKVJ

A NOTE ABOUT THE AUTHOR

B.J. Condrey was born in Winnsboro, Texas. Married to Allison, they have a son named Ezra. His educational background consists of the following:

B.A. Psychology
University of Missouri-Kansas City

B.A. Philosophy
University of Missouri-Kansas City

M.A. Philosophy
University of Southern Mississippi

B.J. served as a staff pastor in various roles (youth, college, small group, hospital visitation) at Grace Fellowship in Winnsboro, Texas and then at Resurrection Life in Picayune, Mississippi. After serving on staff as a pastor in the local church for over ten years, he entered the mission field of philosophy. He has taught philosophy at Pearl River Community College, Spokane Falls Community College, Whitworth University, and Gonzaga University. He will begin working on his PhD in *Christian Ethics and Practical Theology* in September 2017 at the University of Edinburgh where he was recently awarded a scholarship.

He has three other books available on Amazon in Kindle format and paper format—*Where Does God Go, The Word As A Vehicle,* and *Breaking Ground.*

111

In addition, you can follow his blog at www.savethechristians.org.